Medical Genetics for the Modern Clinician

Medical Genetics
for the Modern Clinician

Judith A. Westman, MD

Fellow, American College of Medical Genetics

Fellow, American Association of Pediatrics

Associate Professor, Clinical Internal Medicine

Associate Dean for Student Affairs and Medical Education Administration

The Ohio State University College of Medicine and Public Health

Columbus, Ohio

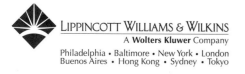

LIPPINCOTT WILLIAMS & WILKINS
A **Wolters Kluwer** Company
Philadelphia • Baltimore • New York • London
Buenos Aires • Hong Kong • Sydney • Tokyo

Acquisitions Editor: Betty Sun
Managing Editor: Crystal Taylor
Marketing Manager: Joseph Schott
Production Editor: Jennifer D. Glazer
Designer: Doug Smock
Compositor: Maryland Composition
Printer: Courier Westford

351 West Camden Street
Baltimore, Maryland 21201-2436 USA

530 Walnut Street
Philadelphia, Pennsylvania 19106-3621 USA

Printed in the United States of America

Library of Congress Cataloging-in-Publication Data
Westman, Judith A.
  Medical genetics for the modern clinician / Judith A. Westman.
      p. ; cm.
  ISBN 0-7817-5760-6
  1. Medical genetics. I. Title. [DNLM: 1. Genetics, Medical.]
RB155.W43 2006
616′.042—dc22

                              2005002003

The publishers have made every effort to trace the copyright holders for borrowed material. If they have inadvertently overlooked any, they will be pleased to make the necessary arrangements at the first opportunity.

To purchase additional copies of this book, call our customer service department at **(800) 638-3030** or fax orders to **(301) 824-7390**. International customers should call **(301) 714-2324**.

Visit Lippincott Williams & Wilkins on the Internet: http://www.lww.com. Lippincott Williams & Wilkins customer service representatives are available from 8:30 am to 6:00 pm, EST, Monday through Friday.

05 06 07 08 09
1 2 3 4 5 6 7 8 9 10

Dedication

To my husband of 25 years, Dave, and the patience he has exhibited

To our four clones—Matt, Joel, Rachel, and Debbie—and their good humor

*To my father, Paul M. Whetstone, MD, for the daily common sense he showed
in a small town family practice and taught to me*

*To my mother, Anna M. Whetstone, MD, as a wife and mother of four,
for her thirst for knowledge and excellence and for her pioneering spirit as a
woman in medicine in a small town family practice*

Faculty Resources

Ancillary content is available online to adopting instructors. The Web site includes critical thinking, ethical issues extension, and team learning exercises; case studies and discussions; bibliographies; and downloadable files of figures, including color versions of photographs and figures not found in this book. For more information and to obtain access to the faculty resources Web site, please contact your local sales representative or visit http://connection.lww.com. To locate your representative, visit http://lww.com/replocator/map.

Preface

As a teacher of genetics to medical students and a practitioner of clinical genetics for 17 years, I have found it exciting to see the steady incorporation of clinical genetics into almost all medical specialties. Clinical genetics used to be limited to pediatrics and the maternal–fetal medicine subspecialty of obstetrics. It has now spread to specialties dealing with adult-onset disorders, particularly in internal medicine, neurology, surgery, gynecology, and ophthalmology. Within the very broad specialty of internal medicine, clinical genetics has practical clinical significance in hematology, oncology, cardiology, gastroenterology, pulmonology, and endocrinology. New advances are announced weekly in scientific and lay literature. Clinical genetics is an area with rapid "translational" value whose new discoveries in the laboratory are rapidly translated to practical use with actual patients.

As the field of clinical genetics has expanded, medical student education has also dramatically changed. Quarter- or semester-long courses in specific disciplines are rarely taught now. Instead, modular courses with integration of discipline-specific topics into organ-specific multidisciplinary blocks have been created. In addition to integration of the curriculum, teaching methods have changed. Large group lecture–based sessions are reduced in frequency, with a shift to an emphasis on small-group sessions involving techniques such as team-based learning, case-based instruction, and exercises intended to promote critical thinking and problem-solving skills. While the faculty work to incorporate these pedagogical techniques, students look ahead to their clinical years and the knowledge needed to care for patients. Medical students are also obsessed with the looming administration of the United States Medical Licensing Examination (USMLE) Step 1 at the end of their preclinical years. Therefore, all course material is judged by two questions: (*a*) What does this have to do with practicing medicine? (*b*) Will this be on Step 1? The order of the questions may even be reversed in the minds of many students.

Medical Genetics for the Modern Clinician is targeted to the first- or second-year medical student in a modular integrated course with approximately 2 to 3 weeks for the medical genetics portion. The approach in this text has been to start with a molecular discussion of inheritance, because classical mendelian genetics simplifies the concepts to a point that may no longer be applicable. Each chapter is accompanied by a few USMLE-style questions and a series of pedagogical exercises to assist the faculty. The focus is on the integration of basic sciences (particularly cell biology and biochemistry) with genetics, progressing to the integration of genetics with the practice of clinical medicine.

This book is not intended to provide an exhaustive coverage of all things genetic. The introductory section provides a discussion of genetics in the practice of medicine (Chapter 1) and a very basic review of DNA structure and function (Chapter 2). The middle section contains a series of chapters with scientific concepts, illustrative disorders, and clinical issues that are encountered in medical practice. The chapters in this section progress from commonly used topics (Cytogenetics, Chapter 3; Mendelian Inheritance, Chapter 6; and Cancer Genetics, Chapter 8) to emerging topics (Complex Diseases, Chapter 9; and Developmental Genetics, Chapter 10). The final section looks into the future of genetics in medicine to topics that may be useful in the near future (Individualized Medicine, Chapter 11; and Gene Therapy, Chapter 12). Noticeably absent are entire chapters on topics such as population genetics, immunogenetics, evolutionary genetics, and general molecular genetic techniques, all of which are worthy topics but at present lack clinical significance for the practicing physician. Instead, you will find smaller sections woven into the general discussion. While historical contributions of scientists and previously used techniques are important, they no longer have practical meaning to the modern clinician and have not been included.

Other textbooks discuss the science of genetics in the bulk of the text and incorporate chapters on counseling and ethics at the end. Counseling, risk assessment, and testing issues are included throughout *Medical Genetics for the Modern Clinician* in context with the issue being presented. Each chapter features an ethical issue related to the contents of that chapter; the ethical issue is frequently a common counseling dilemma. These are not the only ethical issues or dilemmas generated by the topic but are chosen to initiate discussion and to keep the student clinician mindful of the patient-centered qualities that should be at the heart of the practice of medicine. The translational nature of medical genetics should always make us ask, "Just because I *can* do something, *should* I?"

The nomenclature of genetics is used throughout the text with numerical designations for chromosomal locations, international standards for gene names, and various designations for mutations found in genes. Human gene names are indicated in italic capital letters; the protein products are in roman capital letters. Genes from other organisms are italic but with an initial capital letter followed by lowercase letters.

The medical students of The Ohio State University College of Medicine and Public Health must be thanked for tolerating my experimentation in the classroom. Their candid feedback and comments have been invaluable in the creation of this medical genetics curriculum.

Judy Westman, MD

Contents

Genetics in the Practice of Medicine

"Unfortunately, most medical schools did not anticipate the changes that molecular genetics would bring to modern medicine. As a result, the ranks of medical geneticists are sparse, and many physicians struggle with the new biology. Furthermore, the nation's battalion of genetic counselors has never grown to the size that would be needed in order to compensate for these deficiencies. As a result, doctors, nurses, and the public will have to do some work on their own to learn about the genes and genomes that will progressively change medical practice."

HAROLD VARMUS, MD, PHD
Nobel Prize in Medicine (1989) for his work in oncogenes
Director, National Institutes of Health, 1993–1999
New England Journal of Medicine, November 7, 2002

FROM GENETICS TO GENOMICS

Individuals born with unusual physical features have been documented in art and literature since Egyptian times. Twentieth century medical genetics, which began in 1902, when Archibald Garrod initiated his study of inborn errors of metabolism, developed from the study of individuals with rare disorders caused by germline defects in single genes. Most of the observed disorders and the newly identified inborn errors of metabolism were associated with severe constellations of symptoms (phenotypes) that affected embryos, neonates, and children. Medical geneticists began to characterize the physical and biochemical phenotypes systematically and to develop theories regarding their causes. Gregor Mendel's theorems from the mid-1800s provided a foundation. Some individuals developed social policies that attempted to limit the impact on the society as a whole of individuals with these unique phenotypes—policies that included institutionalization, forced sterilization, and in Nazism, extermination.

Other than in pediatrics or obstetrics, a medical practitioner had very little reason to learn about syndromes besides cystic fibrosis or sickle cell anemia, because the reported incidence was 1 in 100,000 or 1 in 1 million, and the likelihood of survival to adulthood was limited. A clinical geneticist would be available in most tertiary care pediatric centers to assist in the diagnosis and care of children with dysmorphic features or obvious biochemical disorders. Medical practitioners accepted that disorders caused by single genes might have numerous clinical presentations and compensated by concentrating on the classic presentation of certain diseases.

Molecular Genetics

The age of molecular genetics began in 1953, when Watson and Crick announced their discovery of the double-helical structure of DNA. Researchers then established the connection between the DNA code and protein structure and eventually determined the correct number of human chromosomes, which allowed the analysis of large strands of DNA in the form of chromosomes. This revealed the underlying cause of many birth defects and disorders associated with developmental delay and mental retardation.

An explosion of discoveries occurred in the 1970s, enabling geneticists to manipulate fragments of DNA within cells, to identify specific genes and their locations within the chromosomes, and laboriously and expensively to sequence portions of DNA. Scientists were concerned that this ability to manipulate the code of life would be accompanied by misuse and abuse. Society and the press were caught off guard by these discoveries. A moratorium on genetic manipulation took place until a consensus could be reached among the scientists and the governmental agencies in the full light of public scrutiny.

The first human disease genes were located by brute force and serendipity in the 1980s. Huntington disease was localized to chromosome 4 in 1983 and cystic fibrosis to chromosome 7 in 1985. Two genes were localized to specific regions of the X chromosome in 1984 (Duchenne muscular dystrophy) and 1986 (chronic granulomatous disease). Finding the approximate location is one step; determining the exact sequence of the genetic code is another. The code for cystic fibrosis was identified in 1987, but it was not until 1993 that the full sequence for Huntington disease was known. Scientists realized that these new molecular technologies had an amazing capability to unlock knowledge of normal cellular processes, disease processes, and new therapeutic modalities.

Human Genome Project

The Human Genome Project (HGP), an international effort to unlock the human genome systematically, began officially in 1990 after several years of planning and preparation. Some people hailed it as a $3 billion boondoggle. The first, unglamorous, phase was to develop the technology necessary to allow scientific discovery to occur. The next phase was to find a series of unique segments of DNA spread throughout the human genetic material that would serve as mileposts, a "map" of human DNA. The final phase was to find the exact sequence of the human genetic code. Completion of the final phase was announced on April 14, 2003, 2 years earlier than planned and under budget. The postgenomic era began almost exactly 50 years after the initial publication of Watson and Crick's discovery (Fig. 1.1).

At the same time that the technological and scientific effort of the HGP was occurring, a concerted effort to address the ethical, legal, and social issues (ELSI) associated with the new advances was under way. Earlier efforts in genetics had taught us that these issues must be addressed throughout the process, not as an afterthought. Individuals must be prepared for new scientific discoveries. Issues of confidentiality and discrimination in insurance, employment, and provision of medical care that have not previously been considered are worthy of our attention. Researchers and clinicians need to understand that if they do not address ELSI, they must accept what is handed down to them by others.

Consequences of the Human Genome Project

Society did not have to wait for the completion of the HGP to begin to benefit from its byproducts. The view of genetic disorders began to change in the 1990s as knowledge expanded. The ability to study the molecular and cellular biology of cancer more clearly showed that the genetics of cell cycle control and the development of cancer were linked. Cancer is a genetic disorder but based primarily on acquired genetic changes in somatic cells; only 5 to 10% of cancer cases are caused by inherited germ line genetic changes. Genetics began to influence medical management, surgical treatment, and pharmacological choices in adults. Geneticists had to learn how genes interacted with genetic transcription mechanisms and other processes within the cell, and medical practitioners who had been concerned primarily with physiological processes now had to learn about cell

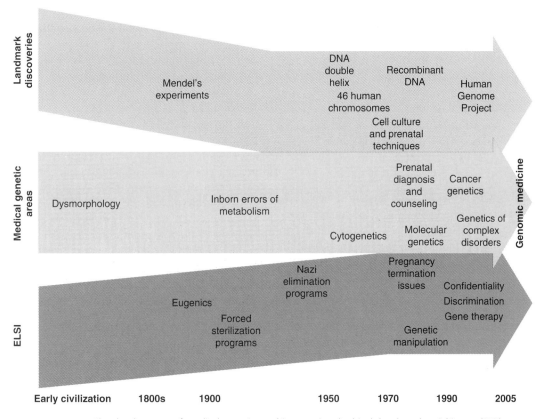

FIGURE 1.1 The development of medical genetics and its associated ethical, legal, and social issues (ELSI).

biology and genetics. Medical genetics entered the consciousness of hematologists, oncologists, gastroenterologists, surgeons, and pathologists.

The HGP has established the number of human genes at 30,000 to 35,000—a number much less than the 100,000 once hypothesized. However, novel processing methods allow some genes to produce multiple protein products, making the total number of genes more in keeping with the original hypothesized number. The dogma of "one gene, one protein" established at the beginning of the DNA era is too simplistic. In the late 1970s, medical students were not yet routinely taught about elements of gene organization, such as exons (expressed sequences) and introns (intervening sequences). Introns and areas of DNA outside of genes were frequently referred to as unimportant "junk" DNA. In this first decade of the twenty-first century, geneticists know that the vast areas of DNA

outside the exons contain regions that control DNA expression in different tissues and at different times in the development of the organism. Many other functions will undoubtedly be discovered. The half-life of medical knowledge has been dramatically shortened in large part because of the HGP. Half of the knowledge acquired by a student in medical school can now be expected to be out of date within 5 years in large part because of the HGP, greatly amplifying the need for medical practitioners to be engaged in lifelong learning. Continued education has always been an important tenet of the medical profession. The modern clinician has a duty to develop a functional understanding of genomics, to apply genomics to preventive medicine and medical therapy, and to learn about associated ELSIs.

Genetics can be viewed as the study of single genes and their functions. Medical genetics has moved from subjective diagnosis by experts based on the study of unusual features (dysmorphology) to factual diagnoses by scientists based on molecular genetic analysis. Genomics is the study of the functions and interactions of all of the genes in the genome with each other, intracellular proteins, and environmental factors.

GENETICS AND PREVENTIVE MEDICINE

Before molecular technologies became available, prevention in medical genetics was limited to two principal areas. One area is newborn screening, which is used to test for inborn errors of metabolism in newborns. If specific errors are identified, a modified diet may be initiated to prevent irreversible neurological symptoms in an affected infant. As a result, phenylketonuria (PKU), an autosomal recessive disorder characterized by a deficiency in the amino acid phenylalanine hydroxylase, has almost disappeared as a cause of mental retardation and developmental delay in children. Women with PKU are now able to survive to adulthood with normal mental functioning, capable of reproduction. However, if the woman no longer follows a modified diet, she will have an abnormal level of metabolites in her bloodstream toxic to the developing embryo. The fetus has a high likelihood of mental retardation, microcephaly, congenital heart disease, and intrauterine growth retardation. A woman with PKU who adheres to a modified diet before conception and throughout pregnancy, however, maintains a normal level of metabolites in her bloodstream and is able to have a normal child. Our success in preventing one source of mental retardation inadvertently permitted another source to develop.

The other area of prevention in medical genetics is additional affected children in a family with a child who has an inherited disease. Parents with an increased risk may decide not to have additional children or to adopt, whereas others decide to conceive and have prenatal diagnostic studies performed on the developing embryo or fetus. They face the choice between terminating and continuing the pregnancy.

The impact of HGP on preventive medicine will be profound. The potential to characterize common genetic variants at multiple locations may eventually allow geneticists to predict the risk of various diseases, even considering external nongenetic factors. Individualized risk assessments may permit the development of prevention strategies prior to the development of symptoms—initiation of specific medical screening tests, lifestyle changes, diet or dietary supplements, or medications designed to prevent or delay the onset of symptoms.

Francis Collins, the director of the National Human Genome Research Institute and leader of the Human Genome Project for the National Institutes of Health, has described a fictitious clinical scenario. In 2010, a 23-year-old man meets with his health care provider and undergoes a number of genetic tests because he has a high cholesterol level and a paternal history of early-onset myocardial infarction. The tests show that he has genes associated with an increased risk of cardiovascular disease and colon and lung cancer (Table 1.1). His physician initiates a personalized treatment plan, which includes drugs to reduce cholesterol level that are specifically matched to the man's peculiar combination of gene variants, early initiation of colonoscopy at 45 years of age, and enrollment in a smoking cessation program. This management plan is admirable, but with our current level of knowledge, such genetic test batteries are unjustified. This combination of gene tests lacks predictive value. However, several of these tests are marketed directly to the public on the Internet.

ETHICAL ISSUES IN MEDICAL GENETICS

Clinicians should be aware of the classic principles of bioethics—autonomy, beneficence, nonmaleficence, and justice (Box 1.1). Bioethical principles are derived from the societal values in the culture in which they originated. The principles used in the United States, Canada, Australia, and Europe are generally derived from a Judeo-Christian value system. Individuals from other cultures

TABLE 1.1 RESULTS OF GENETIC TESTING IN A HYPOTHETICAL PATIENT IN 2010

Relative risk is an epidemiologic measure used to quantify the association between either the presence of a susceptibility gene or an environmental agent and a disease phenotype. It is the ratio of incidence of disease in exposed individuals to the incidence of disease in unexposed individuals. A relative risk of 0.4 implies a person has 40% less risk than a normal person. A relative risk of 4 implies that a person has 4 times as much risk as a normal person has.

CONDITION	GENES INVOLVED	RELATIVE RISK	LIFETIME RISK (%)
Decreased risk			
Prostate cancer	*HPC1, HPC2, HPC3*[a]	0.4	7
Alzheimer disease	*APOE, FAD3, XAD*[b]	0.3	10
Increased risk			
Coronary artery disease	*APOB, CETP*[c]	2.5	70
Colon cancer	*FCC4, APC*[d]	4	23
Lung cancer	*NAT2*[e]	6	40

[a]*HPC1, HPC2,* and *HPC3* are the three genes for hereditary prostate cancer.
[b]*APOE* is the gene for apolipoprotein E, and *FAD3* and *XAD* are hypothetical genes for familial Alzheimer dementia.
[c]*APOB* is the gene for apolipoprotein B, and *CETP* is the gene for cholesteryl ester transfer protein.
[d]*FCC4* is the hypothetical gene for familial colon cancer, and *APC* is the gene for adenomatous polyposis coli.
[e]*NAT2* is the gene for *N*-acetyltransferase 2.
Reprinted with permission from Collins FS. N Engl J Med 1999;341:28–37. Copyright 1999 Massachusetts Medical Society. All rights reserved.

are likely to have a value system that may not emphasize the same principles. Many patients are from Asian, African, and Islamic cultures; therefore, we must be aware of multicultural variations.

BOX 1.1

Classic Principles of Bioethics

- Respect for autonomy
  - Adults have the right and ability to make their own decisions
  - Rights to informed consent and confidentiality
  - Right *not* to know
- Beneficence
  - Act to improve the patient's welfare
- Nonmaleficence
  - Do no harm
- Justice
  - Fairness and equal access to care

Eugenics

Francis Galton, a British scholar and cousin of Charles Darwin, coined the term "eugenic" in his 1869 book *Hereditary Genius*, meaning improving the type of offspring produced. Over the next century, the definition became more specific. The 1987 *Random House Dictionary of the English Language* defines eugenics as "the belief in the possibility of improving the equalities of the human species especially by such means as discouraging reproduction by persons having genetic defects or presumed to have inheritable undesirable traits (negative eugenics) or encouraging reproduction by persons presumed to have inheritable desirable traits (positive eugenics)." Galton emphasized positive eugenics. However, various societies and governments quickly implemented negative eugenic policies for those considered to be unfit. These included prevention of marriage and of racial mixing, institutionalization, sterilization, quotas on immigration, and abortion (Fig. 1.2). Negative eugenics came to a horrible climax in Nazi Germany, where millions of individuals

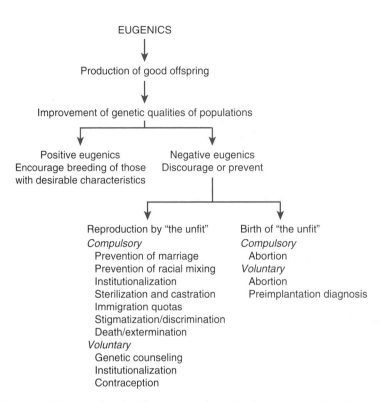

FIGURE 1.2 The conceptual framework and implementation of eugenics in many countries and U.S. states. (Adapted from Epstein, CJ. Is modern genetics the new eugenics? Genetics in Medicine 2003;5(6):469–475.)

were exterminated in the Holocaust. As Nazi Germany embraced negative eugenics, other societies questioned the excesses and bad science associated with it. Compulsory sterilization programs continued in North America and Europe into the 1960s.

The decline of organized eugenics coincided with the rise of the practice of genetics. Although geneticists may bristle at a comparison between eugenics and genetics, there are eugenic issues enmeshed in the practice of genetics, especially in such areas as prenatal diagnosis and termination of pregnancies in which the fetus may be disabled. Geneticists and genetic counselors go to great lengths to provide "nondirective" counseling so that a family or individual receives information about all of the different pregnancy outcome possibilities without judgment or coercion. (Counseling is part of ensuring that an individual is able to give informed consent for any prenatal procedure.) The choice to abort a pregnancy is no longer a societal demand, but the choice still represents a form of personal eugenics. Inherent biases of the health care provider may manifest themselves, particularly in dealing with individuals who are productive in society but who have conditions—deafness, dwarfism, spina bifida—that may be associated with challenges with some living environments. Commonly used terms such as "afflicted" and "birth defects" carry a subtle eugenic connotation. Although medical practitioners may never be able to eliminate all potentially judgmental or biased words from our vocabulary, they must be aware of the effect of their usage on people with whom we interact.

Other Issues Involving Genetic Discrimination

Other ethical issues have emerged in medical genetics. From the beginning of molecular genetic research, individuals have been concerned about the nonmedical consequences of the information generated about the human genome, which has significant implications for individuals, their families, and society as a whole. The most commonly expressed fear is that sharing of genetic information will cause harm. Some sharing of information is beneficial to the individual. It is important that a health care provider be aware of a patient's genetic susceptibility to disease to initiate appropriate screening and management strategies. An individual in an at-risk family may wish to share genetic testing information with a health or life insurer if the test result shows that she does not share the same high-risk genetic changes as other family members. Sharing genetic information is more of a concern when it relates to employment or insurance. Companies may preferentially hire employees with less genetic risk in the expectation that they will have a minimal impact on the company's health insurance premiums or will have less risk of being away from work for extended periods for treatment of a catastrophic illness. Insurers may charge individuals with greater genetic risks higher premiums for health insurance or higher rates for life insurance. To ensure varying degrees of confidentiality, most state governments have adopted regulations. The federal Health Insurance Portability and Accountability Act of 1996 (HIPAA) banned some uses of genetic information for determining health insurance eligibility but placed no limits on premiums. Under HIPAA, an individual with a presymptomatic genetic condition cannot be considered to have a preexisting condition when applying for health insurance or changing policies.

The resultant hodgepodge of regulations provides inconsistent protection across the country. In October 2003, the U.S. Senate unanimously passed the Genetic Information Nondiscrimination Act. A statement in support of the act released by the president's Office of Management and Budget states, "The Act would bar health insurers from denying coverage to a healthy individual or charging the person higher premiums based solely on a genetic predisposition to developing a disease in the future. The bill also would prohibit employers

from using individuals' genetic information when making hiring, firing, job placement, or promotion decisions. .. Unwarranted use of genetic information, and the fear of potential discrimination, threatens both society's ability to use new genetic technologies to improve human health and the ability to conduct the very research needed to understand, treat, and prevent diseases." The U.S. House of Representatives did not act on the legislation.

The implications of ELSIs in medical genetics have traditionally been relegated to a chapter at the end of genetics textbooks almost as an afterthought. Clinicians who practice genomic medicine must routinely consider ELSIs, just as they would think about common side effects when prescribing a medication.

USMLE-Style Questions

1. Two medical students marry and are urged by their respective parents to have three or four children. "You're intelligent and will return a lot to society. It's your duty to put more people like you into the world to improve it." Which concept does this example illustrate?
   a. Beneficence
   b. Negative eugenics
   c. Nondirective counseling
   d. Positive eugenics

2. In 1924, Congressman Robert Clancy of Detroit denounced the Immigration Act of 1924, which imposed severe immigration quotas on several ethnic groups. He stated, "Since the foundations of the American commonwealth were laid in colonial times over 300 years ago, vigorous complaint and more or less bitter persecution have been aimed at newcomers to our shores. Also the congressional reports of about 1840 are full of abuse of English, Scotch, Welsh immigrants as paupers, criminals, and so forth...The 'Know-Nothings,' lineal ancestors of the Ku-Klux Klan, bitterly denounced the Irish and Germans as mongrels, scum, foreigners, and a menace to our institu-

tions... All are riff-raff, unassimilables, 'foreign devils,' swine not fit to associate with the great chosen people—a form of national pride and hallucination as old as the division of races and nations." Which concept does this example illustrate indirectly?

    a. Justice
    b. Negative eugenics
    c. Positive eugenics
    d. Respect for autonomy

SUGGESTED READINGS

Clayton EW. Ethical, legal, and social implications of genomic medicine. N Engl J Med 2003;349:562–569.

Collins FS. Shattuck Lecture—Medical and societal consequences of the Human Genome Project. N Engl J Med 1999;341(1):28–37.

Epstein CJ. Is modern genetics the new eugenics? Genetics in Medicine 2003;5(6):469–475.

Genome timeline. What a long, strange trip it's been . . . Nature 2001;409(6822):756–757.

Guttmacher AE, Collins FS. Genomic medicine—a primer. N Engl J Med 2002;347:1512–1520.

Guttmacher AE, Collins FS. Welcome to the genomic era. N Engl J Med 2003;349:996–998.

Khoury MJ. Genetics and genomics in practice: The continuum from genetic disease to genetic information in health and disease. Genet Med 2003;5:261–268.

Varmus H. Getting ready for gene-based medicine. N Engl J Med 2002;347:1526–1527.

WEB RESOURCES

http://www.nhgri.nih.gov OR http://www.genome.gov
    National Human Genome Research Institute.

http://www.ncbi.nih.gov/
    National Center for Biotechnology Information.

http://www.nhgri. nih.gov/10001772
    About the Human Genome Project.

http://www.genome.gov/10001754
    About the ethical, legal, and social implications (ELSI) program.

http://www.nhgri. nih.gov/PolicyEthics
    Policy and ethics: critical issues and legislation surrounding genetic research.

http://www.cdc.gov/ genomics/hugenet
    Office of Genomics and Disease Prevention. Center for Disease Control. Human Genome Epidemiology Network (HuGENet). HuGE case studies combine genetic epidemiology and genomics.

DNA Structure, Function, and Replication: A Review

BASIC STRUCTURE OF DNA

DNA (deoxyribonucleic acid) is a regular topic of textbooks in middle school, high school, and university classes. It is therefore expected that the clinician reader has mastered some key concepts of DNA structure and function. Some key concepts of DNA structure and function are summarized in the following list.

- DNA molecules consist of two strands of polynucleotide chains.
- A nucleotide consists of a five-carbon sugar (deoxyribose), one to three phosphate groups, and a nitrogen-containing base.
- The base may be either a purine (adenine [A] or guanine [G]) or a pyrimidine (cytosine [C] or thymine [T]).
- The two strands are held together by hydrogen bonds between a complementary purine and pyrimidine base. A always binds with T. G always binds with C (Fig. 2.1).
- The molecular structure of the base pairs is planar and represents the rungs of the DNA ladder.
- The nucleotides are linked covalently by phosphodiester bonds through the 3′-hydroxyl group of one sugar and the 5′-phosphate of the next. The sugar–phosphate groups that represent the sides of the ladder twist around each other, forming the double helix.
- The sequence of the nucleotides contains the message, or code, of the DNA. A triplet, or trinucleotide, code is used; different triplet sequences result in the incorporation of one of 20 amino acids into the final protein. Most of the sequence consists of controlling mechanisms and areas that do not result in the production of a protein product.
- The genetic material in humans, or genome, contains approximately 3.2×10^9 nucleotides in each cell.

TERTIARY STRUCTURE OF DNA

The DNA molecule is not simply a schematic diagram of a twisted ladder. We must consider molecules as three-dimensional space-filling structures if we are to understand how they interact with other molecules. The coiling of the double helix creates two grooves, a large or major groove and a smaller or minor groove (Fig. 2.2—see color insert). These grooves play critical roles in the interaction between DNA and proteins that control its transcription and regulation. In the major groove, the space is sufficiently large to expose portions of the sides of the hydrogen-bound base pairs. A particular sequence of DNA bases may attract a portion of a protein molecule that is complementary with the sequence through a combination of tertiary structure of the protein, amino acid side chains, and hydrogen bonding. This recognition of a DNA sequence by a protein allows regulation of DNA to occur. The minor groove plays a similar role, but the amount of exposure is limited by the smaller size of the groove. As such, only small interactions are possible.

DNA molecules are not rigid structures but participate in local twisting, stretching, bend-

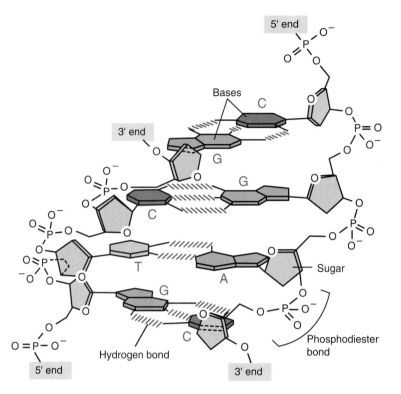

FIGURE 2.1 Three-dimensional schematic drawing of A-T/G-C hydrogen bonding to show planar structure. The purine and pyrimidine bases are planar molecules that form hydrogen bonds between the A-T and G-C pairs; these base pairs represent the rungs of the DNA ladder. The deoxyribose sugar is joined covalently to the bases and with phosphate to form the sides of the DNA helix.

ing, and unwinding of the double-stranded helix. Some sequences create bends or kinks which serve as the recognition site for binding by proteins involved in replication, transcription, gene expression regulation, or DNA damage repair. Changes in the tertiary structure may also be caused by interaction with other molecules, with some binding proteins inducing bends in the helix greater than 90°. Some transcription factors bind far upstream from the transcription initiation site and may cause looping of the intervening DNA, which allows the upstream transcription factor to interact with the transcription initiation proteins at the promoter site.

MITOCHONDRIAL DNA

Most DNA is found within the nucleus of the cell, but a small amount lies within the mitochondria, the cytoplasmic organelles present in variable numbers in all human cells. Mitochondria provide adenosine triphosphate (ATP) energy to the cells through oxidation. Mitochondrial DNA resembles bacterial DNA in the following ways:

- Has a circular rather than a linear double helix form
- Has no unexpressed sequences
- Exists as multiple copies within a single organelle

Mitochondria, like bacteria, replicate by dividing in two. On the basis of these similarities, it is believed that mitochondria are descended from bacteria that developed a symbiotic relationship with cells in a very early era of planetary life.

CELL CYCLE

A DNA molecule must do more than simply carry the genetic code. It must be able to replicate and then separate reliably into daughter cells at each cell division. The cycle of duplication and division is known as the **cell cycle** (Fig. 2.3).

Interphase

The cell spends the longest time in **interphase**, which consists of 3 phases, G_1, S, and G_2. DNA synthesis occurs during the S phase, whereas gene transcription, protein synthesis, and cell growth occur in all three phases. During interphase, individual DNA molecules are not visible by light microscopy, although some genetic material is visible in the nucleolus of the nucleus, a region in which the parts of the different DNA strands that carry genes for ribosomal RNA cluster together. Proteins ultimately combine with the synthesized ribosomal RNAs to form ribosomes.

DNA exists in the cell in a complex with proteins known as **chromatin**. The DNA is tightly wrapped around a disc-shaped histone complex of eight histone proteins: two molecules each of H2A, H2B, H3, and H4. Each histone has a long N-terminal amino acid tail that extends from the package and serves an important role in further control of chromatin structure. Histone function is so integral to eukaryotic cell life that histone structure is virtually identical in all eukaryotes. The wrapped segment of DNA, the histone octamer, and the length of DNA to the next bundle together form a **nucleosome** (Fig. 2.4—see color insert). Nucleosomes exist in chains approximately 11 nm in diameter. DNA material taken from interphase nuclei is typically found in a fiber 30 nm in diameter, thought to be nucleosomes pulled together by another histone (H1), possibly in a zigzag pattern. Additional mechanisms and proteins are responsible for further condensation into the metaphase chromosome, approximately 1400 nm in diameter. The entire collection of DNA and related proteins forms the chromatin.

In an interphase nucleus, chromatin may be in various states of condensation. Regions undergoing gene expression are more extended and are referred to as **euchromatin** ("normal" chromatin). Regions with genes that are

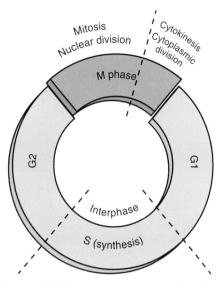

FIGURE 2.3 Cell cycle. The longest portion of the cell cycle is interphase, consisting of G1, S, and G2 phases. DNA synthesis occurs in S phase. Mitosis, or M, phase is relatively short but critical to the generation of two daughter cells.

"quiet" are more condensed. Highly condensed chromatin is **heterochromatin** ("different" chromatin).

The histone tails extending from the nucleosomes are crucial to the regulation of chromatin structure. They are capable of covalent modification such as acetylation by a histone acetylase or removal of the group by a histone deacetylase. The addition of the acetyl group by a histone acetylase alters the chromatin structure, creates separation, and increases accessibility to the DNA, attracting additional proteins. Histone deacetylases remove the acetyl group and make the region less accessible to transcription factors. The deacetylases also interact with other transcription repressors (see Chapter 4). Such activity plays an important role in control of gene expression.

The cell cycle is governed by cyclically activated protein kinases through interaction with protein binders called **cyclins**. The kinases are referred to as **cyclin-dependent kinases** (**Cdks**). Activated cyclins trigger the transitions from one part of the cell cycle to the next. Molecular mechanisms also are responsible for stopping cell cycle progression, but these are less well understood. A specific cyclin–Cdk complex helps drive cells into the mitotic or M phase (M-Cdk). The first visible sign that a cell is about to enter the M phase is the progressive condensation of the DNA material into microscopically visible chromosomes at the end of the G_2 phase.

Mitosis

During the M phase, the cell must separate its chromosomes, which were replicated during the preceding S phase. The chromosomes must be accurately distributed to each new daughter cell so that each receives an identical copy of the genome. When the chromosomes are duplicated in the S phase, the identical copies (**sister chromatids**) continue to be tightly bound in parallel by protein complexes called **cohesins.** As the M phase is initiated, the M-Cdk complex triggers accumulation of protein complexes, **condensins**, onto DNA, which work on each individual DNA molecule to condense the chromosomes progressively by coiling them up. During this initial stage of mitosis or prophase (Fig. 2.5), the mitotic spindle also begins to assemble.

Microtubules that grow out from a **centrosome** outside the nucleus are normally responsible for movement of organelles throughout the cytoplasm. During the S phase, the centrosome replicates just as the chromosome material is replicated. The two centromeres start to move to opposite poles of the cell to form the two poles of the **mitotic spindle**, the mechanism responsible for the orderly separation of the chromosomes. Each centrosome consists of a protein matrix that contains hundreds of embedded rings of **γ-tubulin**, which initiate microtubule growth. One end of the microtubules remains attached to the centrosome, and the other end is free in the cytoplasm. The microtubules are made of α- and β-**tubulin** subunits, which are added or lost in a balanced fashion but are maintained by **microtubule-associated proteins** (**MAPs**). At the start of mitosis, M-Cdk reduces the ability of the MAPs to stabilize microtubules. The normal cytoplasmic microtubules disassemble, and new microtubules that will form the mitotic spindle assemble.

The mitotic spindle must assemble and disassemble for normal mitosis to occur. Some drugs interfere with the balance of micro-

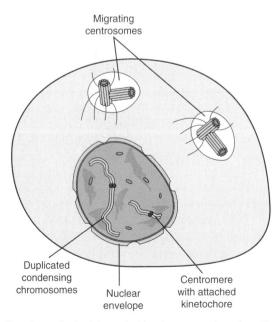

Migrating
centrosomes

Duplicated
condensing
chromosomes

Nuclear
envelope

Centromere
with attached
kinetochore

FIGURE 2.5 Prophase. The first phase of mitosis is marked by chromosomal condensation within the nucleus, migration of duplicated centrosomes, and extension of microtubules from the centrosomes.

tubular growth, either blocking addition of tubulin subunits or preventing them from losing subunits. Either action obstructs cellular mitosis (Box 2.1).

The nuclear envelope breaks down suddenly in **prometaphase** and allows the microtubules of the developing mitotic spindle to contact the chromosomes and bind to them at their **kinetochores**. The kinetochore is a protein complex that assembles on the condensed chromosomes at a constricted region called the **centromere**. (The molecular structure of a centromere is discussed in Chapter 4.) Each pair of sister chromatids has its own pair of kinetochores, facing in opposite

directions, which promote linkage to microtubules extending from the two centrosomes moving into position at opposite ends of the cell. Between 20 and 40 microtubules bind to each human kinetochore (Fig. 2.7).

Abnormal functioning of the kinetochore is involved in human disease. The protein product of the *APC* gene (named for its association with adenomatous polyposis coli, another name for familial adenomatous polyposis; see Chapter 8) normally associates with the cytoplasmic end of microtubules and facilitates the connection with the kinetochore. In cancer cells, acquired mutations in the microtubule-binding portion of *APC* are associated with

BOX 2.1

Drugs That Obstruct Mitosis

Colchicine is an anti-inflammatory drug historically used in the treatment of acute gout and familial Mediterranean fever. Acute gout is an X-linked recessive form of arthritis caused by an abnormality in the purine synthesis pathway that results in overproduction of uric acid and deposition of uric acid crystals in joints. Familial Mediterranean fever is an autosomal recessive disorder with a 1 in 3 to 1 in 7 carrier rate among North African Jews, Turks, Armenians, Iraqi Jews, and Arabs. Colchicine has been found to bind to free tubulin and prevent its incorporation into microtubules. It is used in the clinical laboratory to prepare cells for cytogenetic analysis by blocking separation of condensed replicated chromosomes. *Paclitaxel* (Taxol) is a drug derived in 1971 from the bark of the Pacific yew tree (*Taxus brevifolia*). It binds to microtubules and prevents subunit loss, although subunit addition continues. The blockage of microtubule disassembly results in lack of mitotic progression and cell death (**Fig 2.6**). Paclitaxel and other taxanes are used to treat metastatic cancers of the ovary, breast, and lung because of their ability to cause cell death in cancer cells, which have a high mitotic rate.

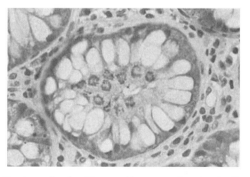

FIGURE 2.6 Mitotic plate. Ovarian cells of a 47-year-old woman diagnosed with ovarian cancer and treated with paclitaxel. Note the uniform appearance of the nuclei, which are all frozen in the middle of mitotic segregation. The chromatids have separated and are being pulled to opposite poles. (Reprinted with permission from Wu K et. al. N Engl J Med 2001;344:815. Copyright 2001 Massachusetts Medical Society. All rights reserved.)

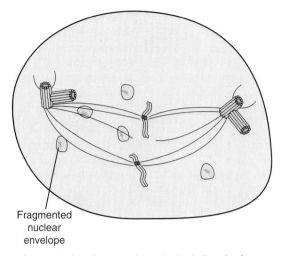

Fragmented
nuclear
envelope

FIGURE 2.7 Prometaphase. A fragmented nuclear membrane is the hallmark of prometaphase. Centrosomes have not quite reached the poles, but microtubules have extended to contact the kinetochores.

abnormal segregation of chromosomes during mitosis. Systemic sclerosis, also known as scleroderma, is an autoimmune disorder in which antibodies attack components of an individual's own intracellular protein machinery, including the centromere/kinetochore complex, DNA topoisomerase I, and nucleolar proteins such as RNA polymerase I. The CREST subset of systemic sclerosis (**c**alcinosis, **R**aynaud's phenomenon, **e**sophageal dysmotility, **s**clerodactyly, **t**elangiectasia) is noted for development of antibodies to the centromere/kinetochore complex, which localize specifically to the inner table of the metaphase kinetochore and to the heterochromatin of the centromere.

The third phase of mitosis, **metaphase**, occurs when the chromosomes, now attached to the mitotic spindle, align halfway between the two centrosomes, which have reached opposite poles of the cell. Tension exists because the sister chromatids are still attached by cohesins and the mitotic spindle is attached to the sister kinetochores.

M-Cdk also switches on activity of the anaphase-promoting complex, a protein complex that is functional late in mitosis and initiates **anaphase**. The complex indirectly releases a proteolytic enzyme that breaks the cohesin proteins holding the sister chromatids together. With the cohesins removed, the chromatids are free to be pulled by the mitot-

ic spindle microtubules to opposite poles of the cell. Anaphase-promoting complex also adds the small protein **ubiquitin** to M-cyclin, which labels the cyclin complex for recognition and degradation by proteosomes. The inactivation of M-Cdk signals the end of the orderly segregation of mitosis.

Mitosis ends with **telophase** and the reassembly of a nuclear envelope around each group of chromosomes to form two daughter nuclei. After the nuclei have formed, the condensed chromosomes are released and return to their uncondensed interphase state with the ability to resume gene transcription.

Cytokinesis overlaps with the last two stages of mitosis. It is the process of cytoplasmic cleavage that completes the M phase and results in the formation of two daughter cells. The plasma membrane develops a furrow perpendicular to the axis of the mitotic spindle during anaphase. The contractile ring responsible for the furrow is transiently assembled from **actin** and **myosin** filaments, the same molecules responsible for muscle contraction, and is attached to proteins on the cytoplasmic surface of the plasma membrane.

MEIOSIS

The mitotic human cell contains 46 chromosomes, 22 pairs of autosomes and a pair of sex chromosomes. Each chromosome replicates into sister chromatids, and the resulting daughter cells have 46 chromosomes as well. The specialized form of cell division known as meiosis is necessary to produce the gametes (i.e., egg and sperm) for sexual reproduction. An egg and a sperm each contribute half the chromosome material to the newly conceived organism. The normal chromosome number of 46 (**diploid** for humans) must be reduced to 23 (**haploid** for humans) through meiosis.

Meiosis involves a single round of DNA replication followed by two successive cell divisions and can only take place in specialized cells, or **germ cells**, in the ovaries or testes. Male germ cells begin meiotic activity at puberty. Female germ cells begin the first meiotic cell division during fetal growth and complete the second cell division when the

egg is released from the ovary, or ovulated, 10 to 50 years later.

Meiosis is similar to mitosis in many ways, except regarding the behavior of the chromosomes (Fig. 2.8). DNA replication occurs in the same manner in both types of cell division, and the sister chromatids are bound together with cohesins. In mitosis, each of the 46 chromosomes lines up randomly at the mitotic plate. In meiosis, however, the 46 chromosomes are paired at the equator of the spindle. In a woman's ovaries during prophase, all 23 pairs of chromosomes the woman inherited from her mother pair with a similar chromosome (**homolog**) inherited from her father. In a man's testes, a similar process occurs except that the dissimilar sex chromosomes (X and Y) pair with each other.

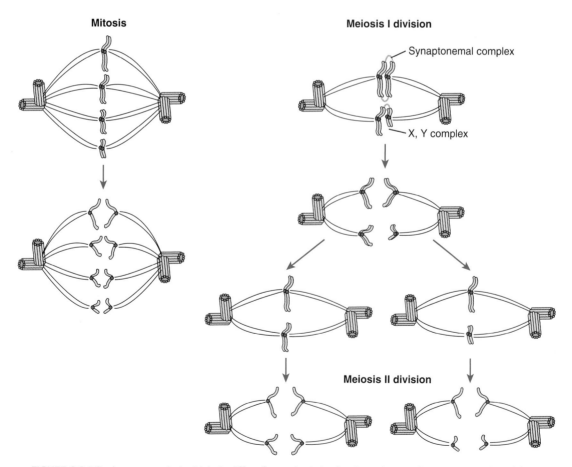

FIGURE 2.8 Mitosis versus meiosis. Meiosis differs from mitosis in that homologous chromosomes pair and form synaptonemal complexes, which facilitate recombination. A second division occurs without additional replication, reducing chromosome material from diploid to haploid.

BOX 2.2

Bloom Syndrome

Bloom syndrome (congenital telangiectatic erythema) is an autosomal recessive disorder with growth deficiency, sun sensitivity, hypopigmented or hyperpigmented skin, skin telangiectasias, cancer susceptibility, and chromosome instability. Multiple chromosomal exchanges are observed in Bloom syndrome cells, almost all between sister chromatids (**sister chromatid exchanges**). The gene that is altered in Bloom syndrome, the *BLM* gene, encodes a helicase whose normal function is to inhibit the exchange of DNA between sister chromatids. When the helicase is not being produced from either *BLM* allele, uncontrolled exchanges occur that may damage normal coding regions, resulting in damage to the cells. (The acquired damage, which results in cancer susceptibility, will be discussed in more detail in Chapter 8.)

The pairs vary in that the maternal or paternal chromosome may be closer to one pole than the other. The exact mechanism for the pairing is unknown; however, the chromosome pairs seem to recognize similar DNA sequences in each other.

The homologous chromosome pairs are held together by a pairing protein or **synaptonemal complex**, which is very precise in its alignment of corresponding DNA sequences on each homolog. The chromosome pairs have already replicated; therefore, four chromatids in each complex are aligned. The synaptonemal complex permits chromatids from each homolog to **cross over** and exchange fragments of DNA sequence. The crossing over can actually be visualized on microscopy. The crossover site is called a **chiasma** (plural: **chiasmata**). This process of **recombination** breaks the double helix on each chromatid, and it must be rejoined. Each pair of homologs is held together by at least one chiasma, usually two or three, which provides structural stability to the pairing after the loss of the synaptonemal complex until the homologs are separated at the first anaphase of meiosis.

Recombination occurs during both meiosis and mitosis. In mitosis, homologous recombination is essential to cell survival; it functions to repair double-stranded DNA breaks and damaged replication forks as well as to create changes in the genome, such as deletions or duplications of regions or conversion of one gene allele to another. In meiosis, recombination is required for structural stability; it also increases the diversity of the resulting individuals (Box 2.2). In meiosis, cohesin joins the sister chromatids together but the chiasmata join the homologs. In the first meiotic division, unlike mitosis, cohesin proteins separate only from the arms of the sister chromatids and not from the centromere. (Components of the first division are designated as prophase I, prometaphase I, etc.) The kinetochores of the sister chromatids orient toward a single pole and act as a single unit, allowing the spindle to pull a pair of now recombined chromatids to either pole.

The second meiotic division, designated as prophase II and so on, proceeds without any additional DNA replication and no significant interphase. The sister chromatids separate to form daughter cells with haploid DNA. The kinetochores function in opposite directions as in mitosis, and the cohesins degrade the entire length of the chromatid, including the centromere.

Random reassortment of the maternal and paternal chromosomes, coupled with recombination between homologous chromosomes, results in the great diversity among individuals, even within the same biological family. If homologs fail to separate properly (**nondisjunction**) or if alignment at crossover is not exactly correct, the conceived individual may have serious imbalances of chromosome material that result in birth defects or death as an embryo, fetus, or infant (see Chapter 3).

Smaller imbalances may affect the characteristics of the resulting individual and his or her offspring (see Chapter 5).

USMLE-Style Questions

1. Sister chromatids are tightly joined by cohesins. Homologous chromosomes are paired along their entire length. Recombination is in progress. Which phase of cell cycle division is described?
   a. Metaphase I of meiosis
   b. Metaphase of mitosis
   c. Prophase I of meiosis
   d. Prophase II of meiosis
   e. Prophase of mitosis

2. The N-terminus tail of the histone protein is able to undergo covalent modification with the addition of an acetyl group. The alteration in tertiary chromatin structure opens the region to interaction with transcription factors. Which of the following regions is most likely to show histone acetylation?
   a. Centromere
   b. Euchromatin
   c. Heterochromatin
   d. Kinetochore
   e. Mitotic spindle

3. Condensins accumulate onto DNA when triggered by a cyclin/cyclin-dependent kinase complex. Cytoplasmic microtubules disassemble and new tubules form from the assembly of α- and β-tubulin subunits. According to this description, which of the following phases of mitosis has been initiated?
   a. Anaphase
   b. Interphase
   c. Metaphase
   d. Prophase
   e. Telophase

4. Paclitaxel binds to microtubules and interferes with the balance in tubulin subunit addition and loss and causes disruption of the mitotic spindle. Which of the following cell types is most affected by paclitaxel?
   a. Bone marrow stem cells
   b. Central nervous system neurons
   c. Mature red blood cells
   d. Outer layer of skin epithelial cells

5. Which of the following disorders involves a defect in the control of homologous recombination in mitosis?
   a. Acute gout
   b. Bloom syndrome
   c. Down syndrome
   d. Scleroderma

SUGGESTED READINGS

Nasmyth K. Separating sister genomes: the molecular biology of chromosome separation. Science 2002;297:559–565.

Page SL, Hawley RS. Chromosome choreography: the meiotic ballet. Science 2003;301:785–789.

WEB RESOURCES

http://www.hhmi.org.
   The Howard Hughes Medical Institute. The biointeractive portion of the site has some good animations and resources. The sex determination section shows recombination and crossing over and their effect on the evolutionary development of the Y chromosome.

Cytogenetics: Microscopic Genetics

Prior to the development of molecular genetics, human genetic material could be studied only by microscopic analysis of the condensed chromatin material present at mitosis. In 1956, after geneticists determined that the normal human cell contained 46 chromosomes, changes in the number or structure of chromosomes were observed in a number of clinical conditions, making cytogenetics the first modern-era technical area of study in medical genetics.

CHROMOSOME MORPHOLOGY, NOMENCLATURE, AND KARYOTYPING

Until the 1970s, chromosomes were classified by size and the position of the centromere. The chromosomes were perceived as **X**-shaped because they were seen at the point in mitosis when cohesin no longer bound the sister chromatids together but the kinetochores had not yet separated (Fig. 3.1). Colchicine is added to the cell culture medium to disrupt the microtubule formation of the spindle apparatus and

facilitate the study of the condensed chromosomes (see Chapter 2). In the 1970s, Giemsa, a DNA-binding chemical dye selective for adenine- and thymine-rich regions of DNA, was used to stain metaphase chromosomes, and a unique pattern of dark (Giemsa positive) and light (Giemsa negative) bands was discovered on each chromosome (Fig 3.2A). **G-banding** is now the standard analytical method in cytogenetics. The light bands, which consist of euchromatin, replicate earlier in S phase, are less densely condensed, are rich in guanine and cytosine bases, and contain more active genes. The dark bands, which consist of heterochromatin, replicate later, are rich in adenine and thymine bases, and contain few active genes. Greater delineation of the banding pattern is possible if the chromosomes are studied at prometaphase, before any separation of the sister chromatids (Fig. 3.2B). Permanently condensed regions of chromosome material at the centromeres, the short arms of the acrocentric chromosomes, the long arm of the Y chromosome, and large regions of the long arms of chromosomes 1, 9, and 16 are made of

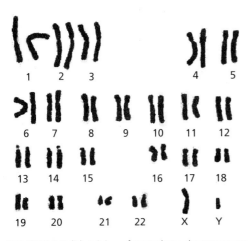

FIGURE 3.1 Solid staining of metaphase chromosomes. Group A (chromosomes 1–3) consist of the largest metacentric chromosomes. Group B (chromosomes 4 and 5) are slightly smaller and submetacentric. Group C (chromosomes 6–12) are very similar and arranged in order of decreasing size, with the centromere moving from metacentric to submetacentric. Group D (chromosomes 13–15) are medium sized and acrocentric. Group E (chromosomes 16–18) are smaller and metacentric. Group F (chromosomes 19 and 20) are even smaller but still metacentric. Group G (chromosomes 21 and 22) are the smallest chromosomes and acrocentric. The X chromosome is very similar in structure and size to the chromosomes in group C. The Y chromosome is similar in size to the chromosomes in group G. (Courtesy of Dr. G. Wenger, Children's Hospital, Columbus, Ohio.)

constitutive heterochromatin and do not contain any genes.

Chromosome morphology and classification are based on the relative position of the centromeric constriction (Fig. 3.3). In 1977, the International System for Cytogenetic Nomenclature (ISCN) established a standard for interpretation of the relative size and position of bands and developed a standard nomenclature and collection of schematic ideograms. Chromosomes are arranged in a **karyotype** so that the shorter arm is oriented upward. The shorter arm is the p (petit) arm, and the longer arm is the q (queue) arm. Locations on the arm are referred to in anatomical language; *distal* is farther from the centromere, and *proximal* is closer to the centromere. Each arm is designated by one to four regions, which may be further divided into subregions. Elongated prometaphase chromosomes reveal additional

subbands, noted by the addition of a decimal point and another numeral, or even sub-subbands, noted by a second numeral after the decimal point. The 1p36.2 region shown in Figure 3.4 should be read "One p, three six point two" (not thirty-six); it indicates the short arm of chromosome 1, region 3, subregion 6, at the .2 subband.

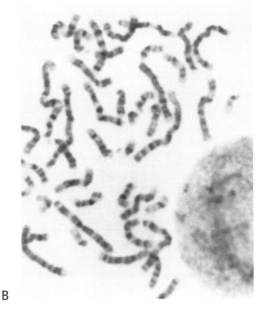

FIGURE 3.2 **A.** G-banding of metaphase chromosomes arranged in a karyotype. Some separation of sister chromatids has started with accentuation of the centromeric constriction. **B.** G-banding of prometaphase chromosomes in nuclear array after disruption of mitotic spindle and lysis of nuclear envelope in the laboratory. The sister chromatids are still bound by cohesin and look linear rather than **X**-shaped. Centromere constriction is not well defined. Condensation has not been completed, allowing higher definition of the banding patterns of individual chromosomes. (Part A Courtesy of Dr. G. Wenger, Children's Hospital, Columbus, Ohio.)

Minor groove

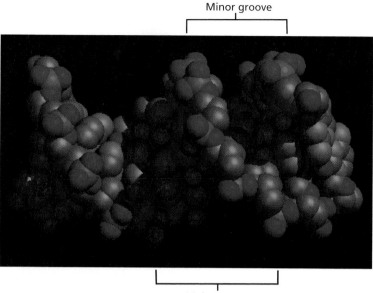

Major groove

FIGURE 2.2 Space-filling model of DNA showing the two grooves in the double helix, which play an important role in the control of gene expression and transcription. (Example from http://www.bmb.leeds.ac.uk/courses/teachers/dnaballs.html.)

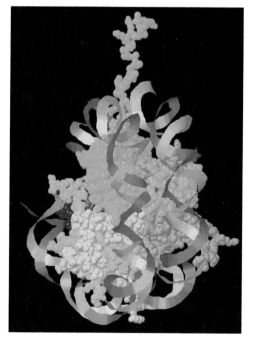

FIGURE 2.4 Nucleosome core particle. The nucleosome consists of eight histone subunits with DNA wound around the proteins. Each histone subunit has a tail protruding beyond the DNA; for clarity, only one is shown in this image. The histone tails are sites of protein modification important in gene control and expression. (Courtesy of Dr. D. A. White, University of Birmingham Medical School, Birmingham, UK.)

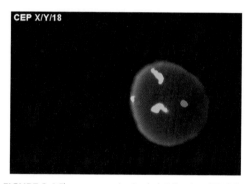

FIGURE 3.4 Fluorescence in situ hybridization (FISH) for sex determination. Blue, chromosome 18 autosomal control; green, X chromosome; red, Y chromosome. (Courtesy of Dr. G Wenger, Children's Hospital, Columbus, Ohio.)

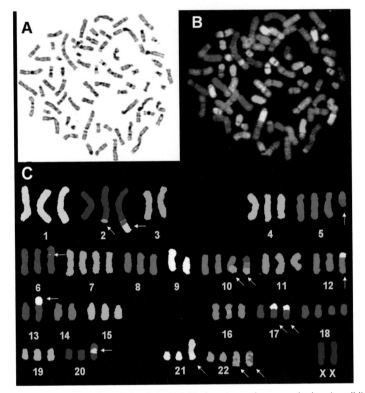

FIGURE 3.5 Spectral karyotyping (SKY) analysis of the K-562 chronic myelogenous leukemia cell line demonstrating a complex karyotype with several structural and numerical chromosome aberrations. A metaphase cell with chromosomes showing (**A**) G-banded pattern and (**B**) SKY display colors. **C**. Chromosomes from the same metaphase cell in SKY classification colors arranged to form a karyotype. Arrows indicate structural chromosome aberrations involving two or more different chromosomes. (Images courtesy of Dr. Krzysztof Mrózek, The Ohio State University at Columbus.)

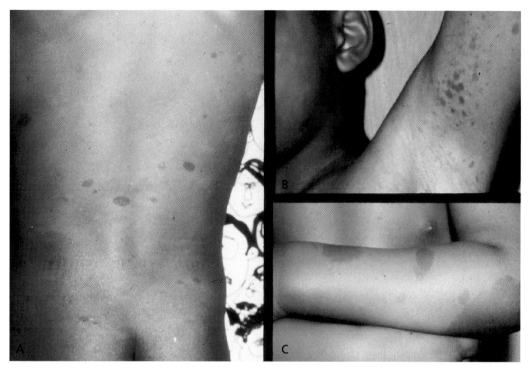

FIGURE 7.2 Children with clinical features of neurofibromatosis type I. **A, C.** Café-au-lait spots, oval lesions with well demarcated margins of varying size. **B.** Axillary freckling. (Reprinted with permission from *Slide Atlas of Pediatric Physical Diagnosis*: Gower Medical, 1987. Image 14.1 from Pediatric Neurology. Courtesy of Dr. M. Sherlock.)

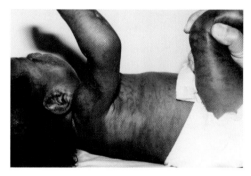

FIGURE 7.12 Infant with incontinentia pigmenti showing hyperpigmented swirly lines following the general flow of Blaschko's lines on the trunk and extremities.

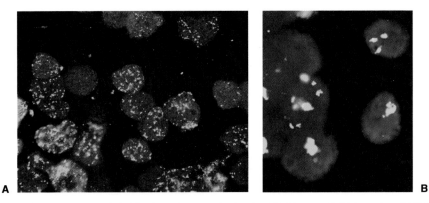

A   B

FIGURE 8.2 **A.** Fluorescent in situ hybridization using a probe for the *MYCN* gene. Multiple copies of *MYCN* in form of numerous double-minute pieces of chromosomal material (green dots). Double minutes are the most common method of *MYCN* overexpression. **B.** Homogeneously staining region in red indicates extensive gene amplification in one chromosomal region. (Courtesy of Dr. G. Wenger, Children's Hospital, Columbus, Ohio.)

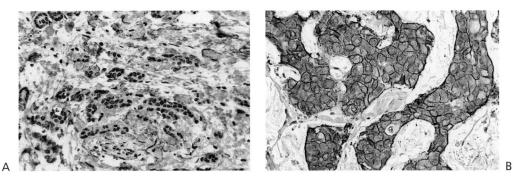

A   B

FIGURE 8.3 Immunohistochemistry of breast cancer cells using a marker for the *HER2* gene product. Immunohistochemistry treats the biopsy sample with antibodies that recognize the HER2 receptor. Further treatment stains the protein-antibody complex with brown color. **A.** The normal tissue shows scattered brown dots. **B.** Cells with amplification of *HER2* have many dark complexes. (Courtesy of Dr. C Hitchcock, Ohio State University Department of Pathology, Columbus, Ohio.)

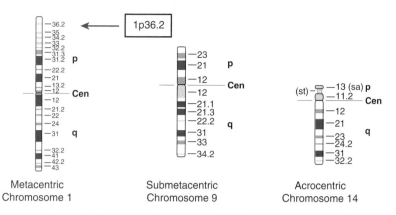

FIGURE 3.3 International System for Cytogenetic Nomenclature (ISCN) ideograms depicting relative centromeric positions of chromosomes. p, petite or short arm; q, long arm; Cen, centromere. Numerical designation of bands begins adjacent to centromere (band 12) and progresses distally to the tip, or telomere.

Banded chromosome analysis may be performed only on cells taken from tissues that are capable of generating mitotic nuclei and are either dividing rapidly on their own or can be induced to divide in the laboratory (Box 3.1). Cells without nuclei (e.g., red blood cells, surface skin epithelial cells) or cells that cannot be readily induced to divide (neurons) are not suitable. Tissue samples are cultured to induce as many cells to divide as possible. The mitotic spindle is disrupted, nuclear envelope dissolved, and stain applied. The analysis is conducted under a light microscope by highly trained technicians under the supervision of a certified cytogeneticist in a CLIA-approved laboratory.[1] Several nuclei must be examined and the chromosomes counted for number and gross structure. A few nuclei are examined in great detail; the banding pattern of each chromosome is assessed and is compared to the ISCN standard. A computer connected to the microscope captures images, and a technician transfers digital images to an organized visual format, the karyotype. The cost varies between $500 and $1000, depending on the tissue type.

TECHNIQUES IN MOLECULAR CYTOGENETICS

Fluorescence in situ hybridization (FISH) combines conventional cytogenetics with molecular genetic technology. It is based on the ability of a segment of single-stranded DNA, or probe, to anneal to its complementary target sequence on chromosomal DNA. Individual DNA probes may be created to target specific genes, or groups of probes may be developed to target chromosomal regions or individual

---

BOX 3.1

Tissues Suitable for Cytogenetic Analysis

Must be rapidly dividing
Peripheral blood (cultured
  lymphocytes)
Amniotic fluid
Chorionic villus
Fibroblast cultures
Bone marrow
Solid tumors

---

[1] The United States Department of Health and Human Services, Center for Medicaid and State Operations, is responsible for administering the Clinical Laboratory Improvement Amendments (CLIA) program to ensure the accuracy, reliability, and timeliness of patient test results regardless of where the test was performed. All U.S. laboratories that conduct clinical testing must adhere to the CLIA quality standards. Research laboratories do not necessarily meet CLIA standards, and test results may need to be confirmed in a CLIA-approved clinical laboratory.

chromosomes. Advance knowledge of the gene sequence or unique sequences in regions of interest is required. Probes are constructed to include or interact with a fluorescent label that can be easily detected visually with a microscope (Fig. 3.4—see color insert). Analysis can be conducted on either metaphase or interphase DNA but may be more rapid if mitosis does not have to be induced. Large numbers of cells can be analyzed with ease, and submicroscopic deletions or duplications can be detected reliably. However, the analysis is limited by the need to know the sequences of interest and the need to develop a probe.

Chromosome painting involves probes complementary to unique sequences disbursed over the length of an entire chromosome, each of which is labeled with the same fluorescent marker color. Metaphase chromosomes are typically used. The technique may detect de novo rearrangements and small marker chromosomes that may be a fragment of another chromosome.

Spectral karyotyping, or 24-color chromosome painting, is the creation of an entire karyotype using combinations of colors in different ratios. Special computer software and analysis are necessary to generate a composite metaphase karyotype image. Spectral karyotyping is particularly useful in cytogenetic analysis of tumors. It is capable of detecting exchanges of DNA between chromosomes but not within chromosomes (Fig. 3.5—see color insert).

Comparative genomic hybridization is used to measure differences in the number of copies of a particular chromosomal segment in two samples. A sample of normal genomic DNA is labeled with one fluorescent color, and a sample from a particular individual or from a tumor is labeled with a different fluorescent color. The two samples are mixed in equal amounts and used as a total chromosome paint to hybridize competitively with metaphase chromosomes on a microscope slide. The samples should hybridize in a 1:1 ratio unless an area of DNA from the sample in question is present in too few copies (allele loss) or too many copies (amplification) (Fig. 3.6). A difference in copy number shifts the relative in-

tensity of the fluorescent dyes from 1:1. The technique is used commonly in cancer cytogenetics and in some in vitro fertilization procedures in the genetic assessment of early embryos (8 cells or fewer) prior to implantation in the uterus. Amplified DNA must exceed 2 Mb to be detected.

NUMERICAL CHROMOSOMAL ABNORMALITIES

Abnormalities in the number of chromosomes have been recognized since shortly after the normal human chromosome complement of 46 was determined. Most numerical chromosomal abnormalities produce a significant change in the phenotype that results in death of the embryo or fetus (Box 3.2). Only a few numerical autosomal abnormalities are compatible with life, unlike many numerical sex chromosome abnormalities, which have a minimal effect.

Numerical chromosomal abnormalities may arise through a defect in meiotic separa-

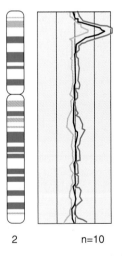

2   n=10

FIGURE 3.6 Comparative genomic hybridization of neuroblastoma tumor demonstrating amplification of chromosome 2p23. The middle black line indicates the 1:1 ratio zone of equal mixing of tumor and normal DNA. If the tumor DNA has more of some chromosomal regions than the normal DNA, the distribution line shifts to the right. If the tumor DNA is missing some of the chromosomal regions present in normal DNA, the distribution line shifts to the left. The ratio is displayed in relation to the ISCN ideogram of a metaphase chromosome 2.

Spontaneous Abortions

According to the World Health Organization, spontaneous abortions (miscarriages) occur in about 20% of all pregnancies. In 12 to 15% of spontaneous abortions, a numerical abnormality has been clinically diagnosed. It is estimated that chromosomal abnormalities cause 50% of first-trimester pregnancy losses but only 5% of pregnancy losses after 28 weeks. Of the pregnancy losses caused by chromosomal abnormalities, approximately 95% are caused by numerical chromosome abnormalities. Between 10 and 20% of the numerical chromosome abnormalities responsible for spontaneous abortions are due to polyploidy. About 80% of the numerical chromosome abnormalities responsible for spontaneous abortions are due to aneuploidy, most commonly a trisomy of chromosome 16 or monosomy of the sex chromosomes (45,X).

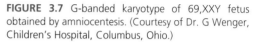

FIGURE 3.7 G-banded karyotype of 69,XXY fetus obtained by amniocentesis. (Courtesy of Dr. G Wenger, Children's Hospital, Columbus, Ohio.)

result in an egg with a persistent diploid state and (*b*) an unreduced number of chromosomes. An egg with the diploid number of chromosomes (46) that is fertilized by a sperm with the normal haploid number of chromosomes (23) produces a triploid embryo.

Most triploid fetuses are 69,XXX or 69,XXY (Fig. 3.7) and are described as digynic (46 chromosomes from the mother) or diandric (46 chromosomes from the father). Diandric conceptions make up 65 to 75% of cases and are more likely to result in a typical early spontaneous abortion; they may develop abnormal placental pathology or *partial hydatidiform*[2] *mole* characterized by focal trophoblastic hyperplasia with villous hydrops along with an identifiable fetus. Digynic conceptions are more likely to result in the very early death of the embryo in the first trimester or the relatively late demise of a well-formed fetus. Rarely, a digynic fetus is liveborn and lives for a few days or weeks (Fig. 3.8).

Aneuploidy

Aneuploidy is a chromosome number that is not an exact multiple of the normal haploid number of 23 (Box 3.3). About 1 in 300 newborn infants are aneuploid. The most common conditions are absence or addition of a sex chromosome and trisomy 21 (Down syndrome).

tion of chromosomes in metaphase or through errors in fertilization. Depending on whether the failed separation occurs in meiosis I or meiosis II, the resulting gametes may have an extra chromosome, may be missing a chromosome, or may have a normal number of chromosomes.

Polyploidy

Polyploidy is any multiple of the normal haploid number of 23. **Triploidy** (3n; 69 chromosomes) is the most common type of polyploidy, occurring in 1% of conceptions. However, triploid fetuses are rarely liveborn. Tetraploid (4n; 92 chromosomes) fetuses rarely occur and are lost at an early gestational age.

In most cases, polyploidy is caused by the fertilization of the same ovum by two or more sperm. The most common other causes are (*a*) errors in meiosis II in the mother that

---

[2] *Hydatidiform* means resembling a watery, fluid-filled sac.

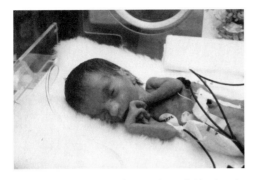

FIGURE 3.8 Newborn infant with triploidy showing extreme growth retardation evident for a term (not premature) infant.

Aneuploidy is caused by nondisjunction (Fig. 3.9). A normal meiosis I division results in the separation of homologous chromosome pairs; one pair of chromosome 3 chromatids migrates to one pole and the other pair migrates to the other pole. In nondisjunction, both pairs of chromosome 3 travel together to the same pole. A normal meiosis II division includes separation of the sister chromatid pairs. Nondisjunction at meiosis II results from the failure of the sister chromatids to separate. The cellular mechanism of nondisjunction may be related to a loss of synchrony of centromeric replication or to insufficient recombination and chiasmata formation.

Nondisjunction is more common in the development of eggs than in the development of sperm. Germ cells increase by mitosis prior to the birth of the individual, but the initiation of meiosis and the length of meiosis are very different in males and females. In males, cells begin meiosis after sexual maturity is reached, and replication of progenitor cells (mitosis) and meiosis continues for the lifetime of the individual, permitting men to retain fertility. In fe-

males, all cells enter meiotic prophase prior to birth and then enter a period of arrested meiosis as primordial follicles. After sexual maturity is reached, several follicles grow further with each menstrual cycle; one oocyte is ovulated each month and several die. Once all the oocytes either are ovulated or have died, a woman enters menopause. One hypothesis is that the length of time spent in arrested meiosis may contribute to the likelihood of nondisjunction; another hypothesis is that chromosomally "healthy" eggs are preferentially ovulated at earlier ages.

Autosomal Trisomies

Most trisomies occur because of errors in maternal meiosis I. Advanced maternal age (greater than 35 years) is the largest contributing factor to the occurrence of trisomies. Figure 3.10 shows the occurrence of trisomy among clinically recognized pregnancies in relation to the mother's age. There is a slight increase in risk among the youngest adolescents, which may reflect a tendency for nondisjunction in the earliest ovarian cycles. As women age, the risk of nondisjunction increases dramatically, and the incidence of trisomic pregnancies increases significantly: 5% at age

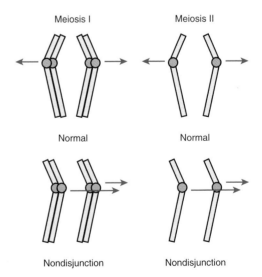

FIGURE 3.9 In meiosis I, homologous chromosomes pair and normally segregate to opposite poles of the dividing cell. In meiosis II, sister chromatids segregate to opposite poles. Nondisjunction may occur at either step but is most common during meiosis I in the developing oocyte.

BOX 3.3

Types of Aneuploidy

- Monosomy = 2n−1 or 45
- Trisomy = 2n+1 or 47
- Tetrasomy = 2n+2 or 48

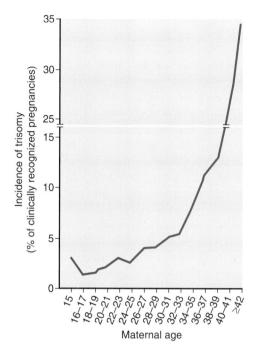

FIGURE 3.10 The incidence of trisomic pregnancies increases significantly with age. Actual liveborn trisomy 21 infants are predicted to occur at 1 in 805 births at age 30, 1 in 365 at age 35, 1 in 110 at age 40, 1 in 32 at age 45, and 1 in 12 at age 50. (Reprinted with permission from Hassold T and Hunt P. Nat Rev Genet 2001;2:280–291.)

30, 10% at age 35, 15% at age 39, and 35% at age 42. The reason for nondisjunction is not known, although there does not appear to be any inherited cause. Aneuploidy in families occurs sporadically; one affected pregnancy or individual does not increase the likelihood of a second occurrence (not considering the age of the mother). Prenatal diagnosis, available for Down syndrome and other forms of trisomy, is discussed later in this chapter.

Chromosomes 13, 18, and 21 are smaller DNA molecules with large sections of heterochromatin. (Fig. 3.2A shows relative size and proportion of darkly stained heterochromatin.) These characteristics may explain the ability of these trisomies to allow a pregnancy to continue to term. Chromosome 21 is the smallest of the chromosomes and produces the mildest phenotype, whereas trisomy 18 and trisomy 13 generate a much more severe phenotype with early death.

Trisomy 21, or **Down syndrome**, is the most common autosomal trisomy of significance in pregnancy and in living individuals (Figs. 3.11). (Trisomy 16 occurs more frequently at conception than Down syndrome but results in early pregnancy loss.) Down syndrome is one of the most common causes of mental retardation. Individuals with Down

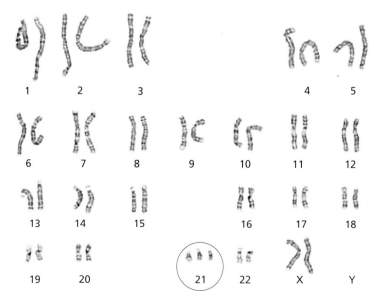

FIGURE 3.11 Karyotype of infant with Down syndrome: 47,XX,+21. (Courtesy of Dr. G. Wenger, Children's Hospital, Columbus, Ohio.)

syndrome have a characteristic facial appearance (Fig. 3.12).

Affected newborns may have congenital anomalies that need immediate attention because of their life-threatening nature (congenital heart disease and anomalies of the gastrointestinal tract) or potential to cause a long-term disability (congenital cataracts). Children are at increased risk for infectious diseases, obesity, seizure disorders, sleep apnea, visual and hearing impairments, hypothyroidism, and skeletal problems, including atlantoaxial subluxation. They have a significant delay in cognitive development with specific deficits in speech, language production, and auditory short-term memory. However, they tend to be cheerful and pleasant in demeanor with fewer adaptive behavior difficulties than appear in other syndromes of cognitive delay. Affected children are no longer institutionalized, and being at home during childhood increases cognitive function. The average person with Down syndrome is able to attend school and achieve at a third-grade level.

Adolescents with Down syndrome may have skin infections, thyroid disorders, and increased weight gain, and sexuality may be problematic. Although females with Down syndrome may be able to have children, they may not understand the cause and effect of human reproduction (i.e., that sexual intercourse produces babies) or be able to use oral contraceptives or barrier methods of contraception independently. Males with Down syndrome may not understand the social implications of certain activities, such as masturbating in public. Specific education and behavioral modification may be necessary. Young adults with Down syndrome are increasingly living in group homes and working in jobs that involve repetitive tasks. They tend to take job responsibilities very seriously.

Adults with Down syndrome may have accelerated aging and an increased risk of valvular cardiac disease. As many as 50% of individuals with Down syndrome older than 50 years of age have evidence of dementia and Alzheimer disease.

Trisomy 18 and **trisomy 13** are the two other autosomal aneuploidy conditions that may be seen in liveborn infants. Trisomy 18 occurs in 1 in 3000 live births. It is associated with severe birth defects that are incompatible with long-term survival. Few infants survive the first year of life, but those who do may be capable of surviving into adolescence (Fig. 3.13). Facial features consist of microcephaly, relatively small face compared to the rest of the cranium, low-set ears, and small jaw. The following features may be detected by prenatal ultrasonography: malformations, which may include central nervous system malformations; congenital heart disease; omphalocele; and hands kept in a characteristically clenched position, with the index and little fingers overlapping the more medial digits. Cognitive and motor development is severely delayed. Children who survive are not able to walk, talk, or feed themselves and require complete care.

Trisomy 13 occurs in 1 in 5000 live births and is even more severe than trisomy 18. Half of

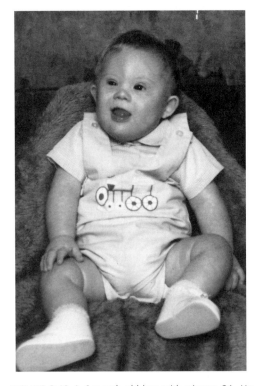

FIGURE 3.12 A 6-month-old boy with trisomy 21. He shows characteristic features of Down syndrome including bilateral epicanthal folds, up-slanting palpebral fissures, small flat nasal bridge, and decreased muscle tone (protruding tongue, delayed independent sitting).

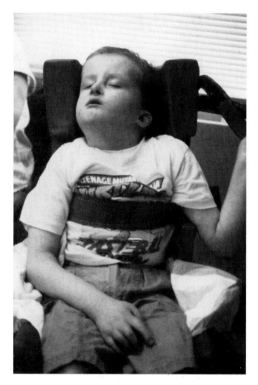

FIGURE 3.13 Child with trisomy 18 who has survived several years. Facial features are petite with relatively small palpebral fissures and a high forehead. (Courtesy of Dr. A. Sommer, Children's Hospital, Columbus, Ohio.)

affected infants do not survive the first month. The facial features are somewhat pugilistic, like a boxer who has gone a few rounds (Fig 3.14). Major malformations are primarily midline and consist of holoprosencephaly (failure of separation of the cerebral ventricles), midline facial cleft, and congenital heart defects. Polydactyly may be present; the extra digit is on the ulnar side by the little finger. Seizures are common, and cognitive and motor development is even more severe than in trisomy 18.

Aneuploidy of the Sex Chromosomes

Sex chromosome monosomy (45,X), or **Turner syndrome**, occurs 1 in 2500 births. (Sex chromosome monosomy should never be referred to as 45,XO. There is no O chromosome!) Individuals with Turner syndrome are phenotypically female, and almost all have short stature and loss of ovarian function.

Autosomal monosomies do not occur in liveborn infants. In general, additional genetic information is tolerated better at the cellular and organism levels than is insufficient genetic information. Monosomy of the sex chromosomes is possible because one of the X chromosomes in the normal 46,XX female is normally inactive (see Chapter 4). Only 50% of cases of Turner syndrome have the 45,X karyotype, with the paternal sex chromosome missing in 85%. An additional 20% have structural abnormalities of the X chromosome, and the remaining 30% have a combination of normal and chromosomally abnormal cells.

Most (95%) 45,X conceptions result in pregnancy loss. The lymphatic system may be obstructed during fetal development; the common thoracic duct fails to empty into the internal jugular vein. The posterior cervical area then becomes a collecting reservoir for the lymphatic fluid, and a large fluid-filled sac (cystic hygroma) may be visible by ultrasonography (Fig. 3.15). The resulting fluid imbalance may be so substantial that the fetus develops hydrops—heart failure, total body swelling—culminating in collapse of the circulation. This is the primary cause of fetal demise in infants who are 45,X.

In some cases, the cystic hygroma resolves and the circulatory collapse is avoided. The resulting abnormality is relatively mild. The resolved cystic hygroma produces a short neck with redundant skin or a webbed appearance, a low hairline at the back of the neck, and low-set ears (Fig 3.16). Hands and feet of affected individuals may be swollen or puffy at birth as a result of lymphatic obstruction. Some girls with Turner syndrome (5–10%) are born with a constriction of the aorta, or coarctation, at the arch, which is also thought to be due to the obstructed lymphatic system compressing the aorta during fetal development.

Most girls with Turner syndrome do not produce oocytes and have poorly formed ovaries (streak ovaries). The lack of hormone production results in infertility and failure to enter puberty. Girls should be treated with estrogen to induce breast development and other features of puberty if menses has not occurred by 15 years of age at the latest. Treatment with

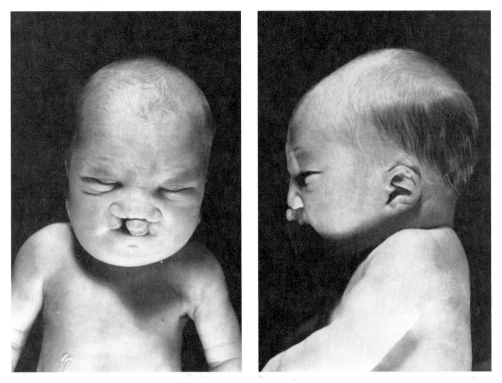

FIGURE 3.14 Postmortem photographs of infant with trisomy 13. Facial features include a slightly receding forehead, a broad flattened nose, bilateral cleft lip and palate, and low-set ears. Compare the coarser facial features with the finer features in trisomy 18.

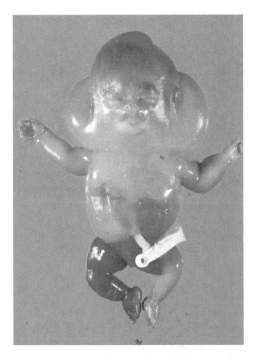

FIGURE 3.15 Fetus with posterior cervical cystic hygroma, hydrops fetalis, and 45,X. (Courtesy of Dr. J. R. Siebert, University of Washington Department of Pathology.)

estrogen and progesterone should be continued to maintain secondary sexual characteristics and to protect against osteoporosis until the usual age of menopause (50 years). Final adult height can be increased by a few inches if growth hormone (GH) is given in childhood as soon as the growth curve declines below the 5th percentile. However, not all affected individuals respond well to GH.

Individuals with Turner syndrome usually have normal intelligence, good verbal skills,

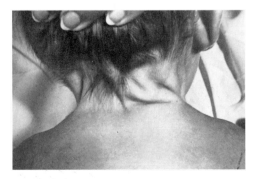

FIGURE 3.16 Redundant nuchal skin and low posterior hairline in girl with Turner syndrome. (Reprinted with permission from Medcom, Inc., from Famous Teachings in Modern Medicine, Human Cytogenetics Part II, 1972.)

satisfactory school performance, and normal peer relationships. However, they may have difficulty with specific visual-spatial coordination tasks and with learning mathematics.

The sex chromosomes may also be present in excess. The most common defects are Klinefelter syndrome (47,XXY), triple X syndrome (47,XXX), and 47,XYY. **Klinefelter syndrome** occurs in 1 in 500 males. The origin of the extra chromosome is maternal in 50% and paternal in 50%. Advanced parental age is an important factor. Affected children may appear normal until puberty, when secondary sexual characteristics may be delayed. The testes fail to grow, testosterone production is abnormally low, sperm formation fails, and infertility results. Some mild cases may go largely unrecognized except for infertility. The recognizable physical features are primarily as a result of the hypogonadism. Testosterone therapy should be initiated at the beginning of puberty to maintain normal male physical appearance and sexual drive. However, therapy does not prevent the infertility. Learning disabilities are common, despite normal or high IQ.

The **47,XXX** and **47,XYY** conditions are unique in that affected individuals do not have a distinctive phenotype. Both conditions are thought to occur in at least 1 in 1000 births. Females with the 47,XXX karyotype and males with the 47,XYY karyotype are usually physically normal, although slightly taller than their siblings, and they may have learning disabilities, although IQs are in the normal range.

STRUCTURAL ABNORMALITIES

Structural chromosomal abnormalities are less common than numerical abnormalities; they occur in 0.9% of all pregnancies and newborns. They are present in 4 to 5% of all men with severely low sperm counts. Structural abnormalities occur in the following circumstances:

- When recombination occurs between nonhomologous chromosomes
- When double-stranded DNA breaks occur within chromatids
- When a centromere pair separates in the wrong plane during meiosis

Reciprocal Translocations

Reciprocal chromosome translocations are common de novo rearrangements that occur randomly throughout the human genome. Short regions of sequence homology occur throughout the genome and permit sequence-specific breakage and recombination between nonhomologous chromosomes, especially in male meiosis. These regions are frequently in noncoding regions of the genome and result in exchange of genetic material between chromosomes without disruption of coding regions or change in phenotype (**balanced reciprocal translocation**) (Fig. 3.17). Balanced recipro-

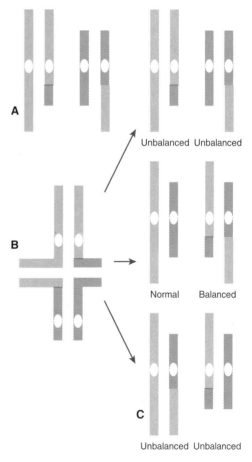

FIGURE 3.17 A. A balanced reciprocal translocation between the q arms of two chromosomes. The karyotype of a man with such a translocation involving chromosomes 6q16 and 17q12 and inherited from his mother would be written 46,XY,t(6;17)(q16;q12)mat. **B.** Pairing of homologous chromosome parts during meiosis. **C.** Segregation options of gametes with outcome in offspring.

cal translocations, which make up most structural chromosomal abnormalities, are present in 3.4 per 1000 pregnancies. Increased paternal age is significantly associated with 30% of balanced reciprocal translocations as well as other de novo structural abnormalities. Phenotype cannot be predicted from microscopic analysis in a de novo translocation because it is not possible to determine whether a coding region has been disrupted. The risk of a serious congenital anomaly is estimated to be 5 to 6% for a de novo reciprocal translocation.

An individual with a balanced reciprocal translocation has an increased risk of having a child with an **unbalanced translocation** because of the possible options of segregation after alignment of the homologous chromosomes during meiosis (Fig. 3.17C). Fortunately, the natural tendency for segregation is in favor of either balanced or normal segregation. An individual with a balanced translocation has only a 10 to 12% risk of having an offspring with an unbalanced translocation. Unbalanced translocations are present in 0.42 per 1000 pregnancies. Small unbalanced translocations involving the subtelomeric portions of the chromosomes are not possible to detect using G-banding alone and require FISH analysis with specific probes.

Robertsonian Translocations

A **Robertsonian translocation**, the most common type of structural abnormality, is a specific type of translocation involving the joining of two acrocentric chromosomes at the centromeres with loss of their short arms to form a single abnormal chromosome (Fig. 3.18). The short arms of all acrocentric chromosomes contain multiple copies of DNA that encode the ribosomal RNA; therefore, the loss of short arms from two chromosomes does not produce monosomy. A de novo Robertsonian translocation occurs in 1 in 9000 pregnancies and carries an estimated risk of serious congenital anomaly of 3.7%. It usually occurs during maternal meiosis. The phenotypically normal carrier of a Robertsonian translocation involving chromosomes 14 and 21 has 45 chromosomes, and the newly generated chromosome is described as a derivative chromosome resulting in a karyotype of 45,XX,der(14;21)(q10;q10).

Approximately 5% of all individuals with Down syndrome have a Robertsonian trans-

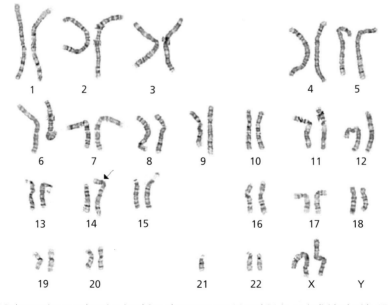

FIGURE 3.18 Robertsonian translocation involving chromosomes 14 and 21 in an individual with 45 chromosomes in each cell. What kind of phenotype would you expect the person to have? (Courtesy of Dr. G. Wenger, Children's Hospital, Columbus, Ohio.)

location as the source of three copies of the 21 chromosome. The most common is a translocation involving 14q and 21q. The individual has one normal 14 chromosome, two normal 21 chromosomes, and the Robertsonian translocation chromosome of 14 and 21. An individual with Down syndrome due to a Robertsonian translocation has 46 chromosomes in each cell; this is denoted as 46,XX,der(14;21)(q10;q10)+21.

Inversions

Balanced exchanges of chromosome material may take place within the same chromosome rather than between nonhomologous chromosomes. Some exchanges may result in an **inversion**, or flipping upside down of chromosomal material. If the breakpoints of the exchange are on either side of the centromere, **pericentric inversion** occurs. The relative position of the centromere may change along with the banding pattern (Fig. 3.19). Some pericentric inversions (chromosome 9 in particular) occur so commonly that they are considered to be a normal variant or polymorphism. Other pericentric inversions create a challenge with pairing of homologous chromosomes during meiosis and may result in chromosomally unbalanced offspring. De novo inversions occur in 1 in 10,000 pregnancies, and there is a 9 to 10% risk of an abnormal phenotype.

If the breakpoints of the exchange are within the same arm, the breaks are next to rather than surrounding the centromere, and

paracentric inversion occurs. The position of the centromere is unchanged even though the banding pattern is abnormal. Individuals with paracentric inversions also have difficulty with pairing of homologous chromosomes; the chromosomally abnormal gametes either have two centromeres or none and are not considered viable. A piece of genetic material that lacks a centromere is lost at the next mitotic division because of failure of attachment of the mitotic spindle.

Deletions and Duplications

Material within an arm of a chromosome may also be lost or added. Lost material may have been from the end of the chromosome (**terminal deletion**) or from the middle portion of the chromosomal arm (**interstitial deletion**). A deletion can affect pairing of homologous chromosomes during meiosis, with the degree of effect proportional to the size of the deletion. Material may be added from another chromosome (**insertion**) or occur as a **duplication** of material normally within the chromosome.

MOSAICISM

Some pieces of art consist of a picture or design made of a number of small pieces of glass or stone, or a collection of small photographs: a mosaic. From a distance only the large design is obvious and not the small discrete objects. Living organisms are also mosaics, with each type of cell a unique object, including possible variation of the genetic composition between some cells. Variation among the different body cells is **somatic mosaicism**. Variation limited primarily to the gametes of an individual without overt expression in other cells is **germline mosaicism**, discussed in Chapter 7.

Somatic Mosaicism

Cells have genetic variation because of errors in cell division or replication, random segregation of mitochondria and their genetic material, or changes in gene expression control. This **somatic mosaicism** is a normal finding in a person but is frequently masked because the phenotype tends to represent the genetic con-

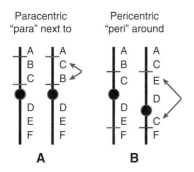

FIGURE 3.19 The two types of chromosomal inversion: (**A**) paracentric and (**B**) pericentric. Paracentric inversions are less common but less likely to develop an unbalanced state in offspring.

stitution of most cells. A change in the genetic constitution may result in major phenotypic changes within the specific cell, and if present in a large number of cells or in critical cell types, it may result in changes in the person's phenotype as a whole. Mosaic populations of cells arise if new mutations that occur early in development do not compromise growth or if new mutations that occur relatively late in development confer an advantage in growth over neighboring cells. Mutations that compromise cell growth early on most likely do not contribute to the mosaic phenotype because the cells do not survive to contribute to the cell population.

Somatic mosaicism of chromosome abnormalities may occur through mitotic nondisjunction (creation of a trisomy) or through loss of an existing trisomy during mitosis (trisomic recovery). Mosaicism for autosomal monosomies is not found because cells do not survive. If the alteration occurs when the embryo has only a few cells, the mosaicism is more evenly spread throughout the body and may be detectable in most embryonic and extraembryonic cell lines and resulting tissues. If the alteration occurs in a cell after extensive differentiation has occurred, the mosaicism may be confined to only one or a few tissues (Fig. 3.20).

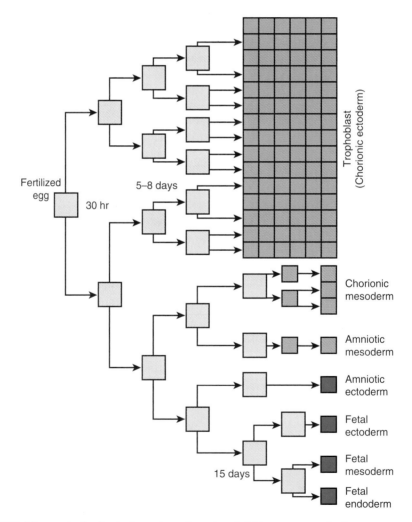

FIGURE 3.20 Cell lineages in the developing embryo. Errors in cell division or gene replication may occur at any point and produce somatic mosaicism in the embryo or one of the extraembryonic tissues. Mosaicism may either be silent or have phenotypic consequences.

Approximately 3% of individuals with Down syndrome have a mosaic cellular composition, with a combination of normal cells and cells with either trisomy 21 or a Robertsonian translocation. The proportion of normal to karyotypically abnormal cells in lymphocyte nuclei may provide an indication of the severity of the phenotype, with a higher proportion of abnormal cells indicating a more severe phenotype. However, lymphocytes do not have particularly important expression value in Down syndrome. The relative proportion in the central nervous system or cardiac tissues may have more predictive value, but these tissues are not used for cytogenetic analysis. The proportion of normal to abnormal usually varies among tissue types (e.g., lymphocytic DNA and skin fibroblast DNA). A mosaic karyotype is indicated as 46,XX/47,XX,+21; the observed frequencies of the different compositions are indicated on the report.

Mosaicism is even more frequent in sex chromosome abnormalities; it occurs in approximately 25% of females with Turner syndrome. Many chromosome combinations are possible. In general, the presence of a normal 46,XX or 46,XY cell line tends to modify the effects of the abnormal cell line and produces a more normal phenotype, although fertility may vary. The presence of 45,X/46,XY mosaicism produces a new phenotype, **mixed gonadal dysgenesis**, which results in abnormal formation of the gonads, with streak ovaries combined with an abnormally formed testis. These individuals have a high likelihood of gonadal malignancy and should have a prophylactic gonadectomy in early childhood.

Confined Placental Mosaicism

Mosaicism detected during invasive prenatal diagnosis may be difficult to interpret. The finding may indicate general fetal mosaicism. However, in most cases, the abnormal cell line represents a chromosomal error that is restricted to the extraembryonic tissues. Mosaicism in the extraembryonic tissues but not in the embryo is known as **confined pla-** **cental mosaicism** and is present in approximately 2% of viable pregnancies. Prenatal diagnostic methods sample different tissues and must be interpreted in light of the characteristics of the tissues and the degree of relatedness to the actual embryo.

PRENATAL CLINICAL TECHNIQUES IN CYTOGENETICS

The invasive prenatal diagnosis of genetic disease has become a routine part of obstetric care. This multidisciplinary process includes obstetrics, ultrasonography, clinical genetics, and laboratory medicine. The goals are to provide choice to a couple at risk for having a child with an abnormality, to provide reassurance and reduce anxiety, to confirm the presence or absence of a disorder, and to provide management options. Indications for prenatal diagnosis include advanced maternal age (older than 35 years), a previous child with a chromosomal or genetic abnormality, family history of a chromosomal or genetic abnormality, and abnormal prenatal screening study.

Amniocentesis

The gold standard for prenatal diagnosis is **amniocentesis** (Fig. 3.21). Amniocentesis has a 0.5% risk of procedure-induced pregnancy loss. Amniotic fluid is typically withdrawn at 15 to 16 weeks' gestation. It may be removed as early as 13 weeks if amniotic fluid volume is adequate and the fetus has shed sufficient epidermal cells into the fluid to permit culture of fetal cells. If inadequate amniotic fluid is present, early amniocentesis may increase the likelihood of clubfoot (talipes equinovarus) in the fetus, most likely as a result of physical constraint from the lack of amniotic fluid.

Amniotic fluid cells are a combination of fetal and extraembryonic cells, primarily from the amniotic mesoderm, amniotic ectoderm, and fetal ectoderm. Fetal cells are shed from the fetal skin and respiratory and urinary epithelia, and they contribute a greater proportion to the amniocytes with increasing gestational age. The fluid itself has an amber color very similar to that of

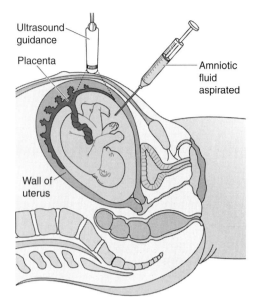

FIGURE 3.21 In amniocentesis, amniotic fluid is obtained using ultrasound guidance. A hollow needle is inserted through the mother's abdomen into the uterus, and amniotic fluid is withdrawn for analysis. (Modified with permission from Willis MC. Medical Terminology: A Programmed Learning Approach to the Language of Health Care. Baltimore: Lippincott Williams & Wilkins, 2002, Figures 15–20*B*.)

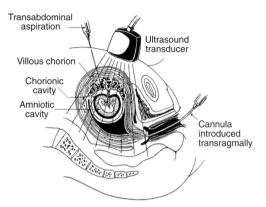

FIGURE 3.22 Chorionic villus sampling (CVS). There are two ways to collect chorionic villi from the placenta: through the vagina or through the abdomen. In the transcervical approach a small tube is inserted through the vagina and cervix and guided to the placenta where a small sample is removed. If an anterior placenta is present, a transabdominal approach may be used by inserting a needle through the mother's abdominal wall in a very similar fashion to amniocentesis. (Reprinted with permission from Beckman CRB et al. Obstetrics and Gynecology, 4th ed. Baltimore: Lippincott Williams & Wilkins, 2002, Figure 24.2.)

unconcentrated urine and in fact is primarily generated from fetal urine. Amniocentesis may be performed up to 36 weeks for diagnostic techniques on fetal cells. After 36 weeks, the fetal cells more completely resemble adult epidermal cells, which are not suitable for cell culture. The amniotic fluid is centrifuged to isolate the amniocytes; these are then cultured to obtain mitotic cells for cytogenetic or gene analysis. The fluid itself may also be analyzed for fetal proteins, which may be useful in the detection of certain birth defects, such as neural tube defects or abdominal wall defects.

Chorionic Villus Sampling

Chorionic villus sampling (CVS) is performed at 10 to 12 weeks' gestation (Fig. 3.22) and has similar indications for use as amniocentesis. The sampled cells are from the chorion, or placenta, and are all extraembryonic in origin (Fig. 3.21). Separation of maternal from fetal cells contributing to the chorion is necessary prior to culturing. CVS has a 0.5% risk of procedure-induced pregnancy loss. If performed prior to 9 weeks, there is an increased risk of fetal limb reduction abnormalities, probably due to disruption of the blood vessels. Confined placental mosaicism causes a 2% false-positive rate, and when it is encountered, amniocentesis is required to confirm the diagnosis. Rarely, mosaicism may develop in embryonic tissues after the extraembryonic tissues have differentiated. This type of mosaicism is not detected by CVS.

Cordocentesis

Percutaneous umbilical blood sampling, or **cordocentesis**, entails obtaining blood from the umbilical cord. A needle is inserted into the mother's abdomen and the amniotic cavity and is guided into the umbilical artery or vein using ultrasound. The procedure is similar to amniocentesis, except that the goal is to obtain blood from the fetus rather than amniotic fluid. It can be performed any time after

18 weeks of gestation but is usually performed only by a maternal–fetal medicine specialist at a high-risk obstetric center. The procedure is associated with a fetal loss rate of 1 to 2%. Fetal blood does not require the same length of cell culture, so cytogenetic results are usually available more rapidly. Cordocentesis may also be used to obtain laboratory measurements to assess fetal anemia and platelet level.

ETHICS Prenatal Diagnosis and Pregnancy Outcomes

There are very few more emotionally charged issues in the United States than abortion, the lay term for the decision to terminate a pregnancy. Abortion pits the right of choice of the adult parent against the right to live of the unborn child. A Google search of "abortion and ethics" revealed 288,000 locations. Individual views on the appropriateness of pregnancy termination are usually tied to the faith-based upbringing of the individual and vary widely in different parts of the world, depending on the prevailing faith and culture of the region. Many individuals use pregnancy termination as a legal method of birth control in case of unplanned or undesired pregnancies. Medical professionals distinguish the different types of pregnancy termination as spontaneous abortion (miscarriage), elective abortion (pregnancy control), and therapeutic abortion (presence of an abnormal fetus).

Prenatal diagnosis of an abnormal fetus, if obtained early in pregnancy, permits the parents to have a choice in the management of the remainder of the pregnancy. Individuals in this situation weigh the predicted problems of the unborn child with the emotional and economic effects on them and their extended family, including existing children. Choices include the following:

- Continuing the pregnancy, knowing that the defect will likely be lethal or that the infant will have significant medical problems at or shortly after birth
- Using the information provided by prenatal diagnosis and choosing to deliver the infant at a specialized facility capable of immediately handling the child's problem
- Using prenatal therapeutic interventions that may improve the outcome and health of the child
- Terminating the pregnancy, a choice that rarely comes easily or without psychological side effects if the pregnancy was planned and anticipated

Two tenets held by prenatal genetic health care professionals are that (a) they should never attempt to influence the outcome of a pregnancy and (b) they should use only nondirective genetic counseling techniques. This philosophy is directly related to the backlash against eugenics and the effort to keep from being labeled as in favor of eugenics. Public health policy makers have occasionally encouraged genetics professionals to use more directive counseling techniques to improve reproductive outcomes in accordance with the goals of public health.

Medical practitioners are entitled to hold strong personal views about the appropriateness or inappropriateness of abortion. Patients are entitled to have all available information about treatment and management options, and practitioners are required to provide the information (informed consent). Practitioners should neither block access to legal health care options nor attempt to coerce patients into a choice of more personal preference for the practitioner. (Cases on the accompanying Web site explore various aspects of physician–patient relationships in prenatal diagnosis.)

USMLE-Style Questions

1. A couple presents with unexplained infertility—four spontaneous abortions and no liveborn child in 5 years. During their infertility evaluation, you suggest that they have cytogenetic analysis to rule out chromosomal problems. Which sample is most suitable for analysis?
   a. Amniotic fluid
   b. Blood
   c. Chorionic villus sample
   d. Gonadal biopsy
   e. Neural biopsy

2. A G-banded segment of metaphase chromosomal material appears lighter than surrounding areas. A fluorescence in situ hybridization probe for a known transcribed gene binds in the same region. This segment most likely consists of which of the following?
   a. An AT-rich region
   b. Centromere
   c. Euchromatin
   d. Heterochromatin
   e. Nucleolar organizing region

3. The q arm of a submetacentric chromosome has exchanged places with the p arm of a metacentric chromosome at a spot near the centromere. There are 46 chromosomes in the karyotype. The individual has a normal phenotype. This rearrangement represents which of the following?
   a. Balanced reciprocal translocation
   b. Balanced Robertsonian translocation
   c. Paracentric inversion
   d. Unbalanced reciprocal translocation
   e. Unbalanced Robertsonian translocation

4. A fourth-grade girl is in your office for evaluation of learning disability. She has recently failed the fourth-grade reading proficiency examination. Physical examination reveals her height at the fifth percentile. Both her mother's and father's height are at the 75th percentile. The girl has a low posterior hairline and shows no evidence of pubertal development. She is quite talkative and understandable. A blood sample is obtained for a chromosome study. Which of the following is the most likely result?
   a. 45,XO
   b. 45,X
   c. 46,XY
   d. 47,XX,+21
   e. 47,XXX

5. During a routine midpregnancy ultrasound, a fetus is diagnosed with a severe congenital heart defect. The obstetrician also notes significant growth retardation and fetal hands held in an unusual clenched position. The placenta appears normal. Amniocentesis for karyotyping confirms the suspected diagnosis. Which of the following is the most likely cause of the abnormality?
   a. De novo paternal structural abnormality
   b. Maternal meiotic nondisjunction
   c. Monosomy of chromosome 18
   d. Triploidy due to simultaneous fertilization by two sperm
   e. Robertsonian translocation between chromosomes 13 and 21

6. A 43-year-old woman is considering having an invasive prenatal diagnostic study. She is at 8 weeks' gestation. Which of the following is the most appropriate reason to select chorionic villus sampling (CVS) rather than other prenatal diagnostic methods?
   a. A CVS sample can be analyzed more rapidly than one from cordocentesis.
   b. Amniotic fluid cells are extraembryonic cells and diagnosis is less accurate.
   c. CVS can be performed at 10 to 12 weeks' gestation rather than at 15 to 16 weeks.
   d. CVS detects open neural tube defects and abdominal wall defects.

SUGGESTED READINGS

Frias JL, Davenport ML. Committee on Genetics and Section on Endocrinology. Health supervision for children with Turner syndrome. Pediatrics 2003;111:692–702.

Hayes A, Batshaw ML. Down syndrome. Pediatr Clin North Am 1993;40:523–535.

Linden MG, Bender BG, Robinson A. Intrauterine diagnosis of sex chromosome aneuploidy. Obstet Gynecol 1996;87:468–475. Contains a good review of current prognostic information for sex chromosome disorders.

WEB RESOURCES

http://www.nlm.nih.gov/medlineplus/downsyndrome.html
Facts about Down syndrome from the National Institutes of Health.

http://turners.nichd.nih.gov/
Turner syndrome. National Institute for Child Health and Human Development, the National Institutes of Health.

http://www.nichd.nih.gov/publications/pubs klinefelter.htm.
Understanding Klinefelter syndrome: a guide for XXY males and their families. National Institute for Child Health and Human Development, the National Institutes of Health.

http://www.marchofdimes.org.
The March of Dimes. Contains fact sheets for professionals on common disorders affecting infants.

http://www.trisomy.org.
Support Organization for Trisomy 18, 13, and Related Disorders (SOFT).

Molecular Genetics: Gene Structure, Organization, and Control

With the development of techniques capable of studying and manipulating blocks of DNA material, the study of medical genetics has evolved from the microscopic world of cytogenetics to the molecular world of individual genes. The basic structure of DNA (see Chapter 2) and its organization into macromolecules, or chromosomes (see Chapter 3), have been discussed. The structure and organization within each molecule of DNA forms the basis for the remainder of the study of medical genetics.

GENE STRUCTURE

Human genes, like other eukaryotes, do not exist as uninterrupted stretches of DNA. The portions of the gene that are eventually translated into a protein product, or *expressed*, are **exons** and are broken up across the length of the gene. The exons are separated by long intervening sequences (**introns**). Introns tend to be much larger than exons and contain critical DNA sequences that participate in messenger RNA (mRNA) processing. Some introns even contain other genes. Regulatory sequences may be present on the same strand of DNA—*cis*—in the untranslated regions preceding the gene (5′), within introns, or even on the opposite strand of DNA—*trans*.

FROM GENE TO PRODUCT

Transcription and Transcription Factors

The promoter region of a gene in the 5′ untranslated region of a gene contains an initiation site where transcription, the process by which the DNA sequence of a gene is copied into mRNA, actually begins. Most genes also have regulatory DNA sequences that are used to switch the gene on or off during the cell cycle, in various tissues or stages of development, or in response to extracellular signals. Regulatory sequences are recognized by regulatory proteins that bind to the DNA and act as a switch to control transcription. These **transcription factors** recognize a DNA sequence because the three-dimensional surface of the protein fits tightly against the three-dimensional surface features of the DNA helix in that region, frequently involving the major groove of the helix. Multiple highly specific protein–DNA interactions occur through repetitive domains within a protein; these include helix-turn-helix, zinc finger motif of α-helix and β-sheet, and the leucine zipper of two α-helices that contains many leucine amino acid residues.

Processing mRNA

The primary transcripts, pre-mRNAs, contain the entire transcribed sequences of exons and introns. The introns must be precisely removed to yield mRNA with the precise code to allow translation into a functional product. The removal of introns is accomplished through **splicing**, which takes place in a massive ribonucleoprotein complex known as the **spliceosome**, composed of as many as 300 distinct proteins and five RNAs; the spliceosome is one of the most complex macromolecular machines known. Once a transcript has been spliced and its 5′ and 3′ ends modified, mature functional mRNA suitable for protein translation has been made.

Special nucleotide sequences span the end of an exon and the beginning of an intron, the end of the intron and the beginning of the next exon, and a region within the intron but close to the 3′ end that provides a site for binding of the intron for removal. These sequences are recognized by small nuclear ribonucleoproteins (snRNPs, pronounced snurps) that cleave the RNA at the intron–exon borders and link the exons together. The excised intron is released (Fig. 4.1).

Changes in the splice site recognition sequences produce abnormal splicing. β-

Thalassemia is an autosomal recessive disorder caused by a defect in β-globin whose gene is at chromosome 11p15.5. β-Globin is one of the proteins of the hemoglobin multimeric protein. Hemoglobin is made of two molecules of β-globin and two molecules of α-globin with a heme group containing iron. Individuals with β-thalassemia have abnormal hemoglobin and chronic microcytic anemia beginning in childhood. Affected individuals require regular transfusions of red blood cells. The β-globin gene contains three exons and two introns (Fig. 4.2). Many of the disease-producing mutations are splice site recognition sequences, which alter the expression of the β-globin protein by variably reducing its synthesis (β^+). Other mutations cause a truncated protein with essentially no production (β°). (See the Web resources for a related case.)

Alternative Splicing

The central dogma of biology was once stated as "one gene, one protein," a concept that has now been disproved. RNA splicing allows more information to be packed into every gene: it permits multiple RNAs and proteins to be produced from a single gene by splicing exons together in different combinations (**alternative splicing**). It is estimated that 40 to 60% of multiexon genes undergo alternative splicing, allowing cells to produce related but distinct proteins from a single gene. One form of protein may be produced in one type of tissue, while other forms are produced in other tissues. This discovery has led to a decrease in the number of suspected genes in the genome from 100,000 to 24,500. The exact number is yet to be determined.

The central dogma of biology was subsequently restated; it maintained that genetic information normally flows from DNA to RNA to protein. We now know that approximately 7% of transcribed RNA is noncoding RNA that is not used for protein translation. Noncoding RNA has been shown to control chromosome architecture, mRNA turnover, and the developmental timing of protein expression. In addition, it may regulate transcription and alternative splicing.

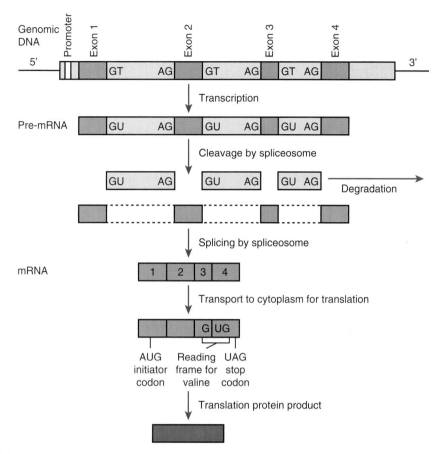

FIGURE 4.1 Genomic DNA contains regulatory sequences, expressed sequences (exons), and intervening sequences (introns). A complex ribonucleoprotein machine, the spliceosome, recognizes and removes the introns and splices the exons together to form the mature mRNA. RNA remnants are degraded. Messenger RNA is typically transported to the cytoplasm for protein translation. The entire length of the mRNA contains untranslated regions in the 5' and 3' ends. The translated protein begins at an initiator or start codon and ends at a stop codon. The triplet codon reading frame is continuous from beginning to end and is independent of the exon/intron junction sites.

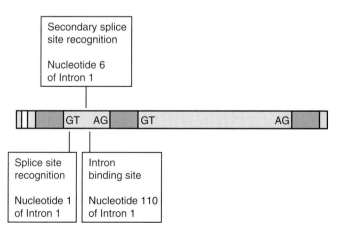

FIGURE 4.2 Common mutation sites in the β-globin gene (1423 bp). Other mutations have been found in the promoter, at each of the exon/intron junctions, and as truncating mutations as a result of the creation of a new stop codon.

Translation

Messenger RNA is transported from the nucleus to the cytoplasm for translation of the genetic code into an amino acid sequence. The triplet code of the DNA and subsequent mRNA is uniform throughout most living organisms; some small differences in the DNA code are found in mitochondria. The site where the ribosome initiates protein synthesis on the mRNA is important because it sets the reading frame for the entire message. Any miscue results in a garbled translation. The eukaryotic initiation site is usually the first AUG codon (coding for methionine) after the 5′ cap of the mRNA (Fig. 4.1) and is read by a special initiator, or start tRNA. The methionine is usually removed later. The start tRNA facilitates the initial ribosomal function. Translation continues until a stop codon is reached (UAA, UAG, or UGA). Translation is controlled by the start tRNA and by regulatory elements in the 5′ and 3′ untranslated regions of the mRNA.

Posttranslational Modification and Localization

During and after completion of translation, the newly formed proteins are frequently modified by the addition of chemical groups to single amino acids (hydroxylation, phosphorylation, and disulfide bonds) or addition of carbohydrates (glycoproteins) or lipids (lipoproteins). The protein may also be cleaved to form a smaller final product. Specific polypeptide sequences that signal a need to transport the protein outside the cell or to a specific location or organelle within the cell may be present; these sequences are usually removed once appropriate localization has occurred. Disruptions in these sequences may prevent the protein product from arriving at its desired location.

For specific details on the mechanisms of transcription, translation, and posttranslational modification, consult an undergraduate text or cell biology text.

GENOME ORGANIZATION

Repeated Elements

No two people except identical twins have the same exact genome. If the DNA between two human genome regions is compared, the sequence is 99.9% identical. Given the size of the human genome (3200 Mb), this 0.1% variation provides many possible genetic differences between one person and the next (3.2 Mb).

Single-Nucleotide Polymorphisms

The most common type of repeated genetic elements is called a **single-nucleotide polymorphism** (SNP, pronounced *snip*). These variations are associated with diversity in the population, individuality, susceptibility to diseases, and individual responses to medicine. This type of variation is particularly noted in the untranslated regions of the genome, that is, in the 5′ and 3′ untranslated regions of the gene, within introns, and in the extragenic regions of DNA, where variations in sequence can occur without as great an impact on function. These polymorphisms are points that differ in nucleotide sequence between one normal person in the population and another. One person has an A-T pair, whereas another has a G-C. More than 90% of all human genes contain at least one SNP, and approximately 3 million have been discovered since the human genome sequence was determined. The challenge is to recognize the few SNPs that are functionally important from those that represent normal variation. The SNP map provided by the Human Genome Project is useful in identifying new genes.

Cytochrome P450 (*CYP*) genes, which have more than 80 protein products, encode a class of drug-metabolizing enzymes responsible for the detoxification of chemicals. The product of the *2C9* member of the *CYP* family hydroxylates about 16% of drugs in clinical use, including the anticoagulant warfarin, the anticonvulsant phenytoin, and the insulin-release stimulator tolbutamide. Impairment of CYP2C9 metabolic activity may cause drug toxicity or inappropriately low drug levels in these medications, which require specific therapeutic drug levels. SNPs in the *CYP2C9* gene determine the phenotype that underlies individual and ethnic differences in drug metabolism. Five SNP variants, which differ by race and ethnicity, produce enzymes with reduced or deficient metabolic activity.

TABLE 4.1 CLASSES OF DNA REPEATED IN TANDEM

CLASS	REPEAT SIZE (BP)	LOCATION
Satellite DNA	100 kb to several Mb	Noncoding
α-satellite		Centromeric heterochromatin
β-satellite		Constitutive heterochromatin of 1, 9, and Y
		Acrocentric p arms and satellites
Minisatellite DNA	0.1–20 kb	Noncoding
Telomeres		All telomeres
Hypervariable		All chromosomes
Microsatellite DNA	<100 bp	Dispersed throughout genome; some coding regions

Individuals who are carriers of one or more variant alleles may be at risk for adverse drug reactions or toxicity when prescribed drugs extensively metabolized by CYP2C9.

Satellites, Minisatellites, and Microsatellites

Sequence variation may also result from variable amounts of repetitive DNA known as **tandem repeats.** Tandemly repeated DNA sequences are most commonly found in noncoding regions and are composed of a repeat unit that is repeated many times within a region. The three classes of tandem repeats are classified by size: **satellite DNA**, **minisatellite DNA**, and **microsatellite DNA** (Table 4.1).

Satellite DNA is usually found near the centromere (Fig. 4.3). α-Satellite DNA consists of 171-bp tandem repeats whose sequences have evolved and diverged among the different human chromosomes. This divergence permits the use of specific fluorescence in situ hybridization (FISH) probes to distinguish between chromosomes. The α-satellite DNA may serve as a binding site for one of the centromeric proteins involved in mitosis.

The shorter minisatellite DNA may be found in hypervariable sequences or at the telomeres. The sequence similarity in hypervariable sequences increases the likelihood of recombination at these sites. DNA profiling

(fingerprinting and forensics) now uses combinations of microsatellite markers for increased ease and accuracy (Fig. 4.4). A single DNA probe creates a complex individual-specific electrophoretic hybridization pattern that is compared band by band for position and level of intensity.

The ends of each chromosome (telomeres) are made of hexanucleotide tandem repeats: TTAGGG in humans. These repeats are repli-

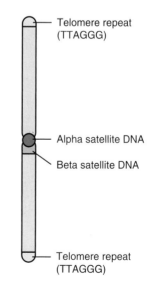

FIGURE 4.3 Location of large regions of tandem repeats. Hypervariable minisatellite regions and microsatellites are more dispersed throughout the genome and are not found at specific chromosomal locations.

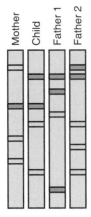

Mother Child Father 1 Father 2

FIGURE 4.4 Use of hypervariable minisatellite DNA in paternity testing. The child will have received half of his or her markers from the mother and half from the father. Which of the two alleged fathers appears to be the biological match?

cated by a special mechanism during mitosis, serve as caps at the ends of the DNA molecule, and protect the chromosomal DNA from being degraded. The enzyme telomerase, an RNA-dependent DNA polymerase or reverse transcriptase, synthesizes the ends of the chromosomes. Telomeres are subject to progressive shortening in the successive mitoses of normal somatic cells, leading ultimately to irreversible growth arrest. If telomerase is abnormally active in a cell, the cell effectively becomes immortal and continues to undergo mitosis. Many cancers are facilitated by continued telomerase activity; therefore, the development of telomerase inhibitors is an important target of cancer investigators.

Microsatellites are small regions of tandem repeats of one to four nucleotides that occur throughout the entire genome and account for 2% of it. Dinucleotide repeats are the most common. Microsatellite repeats within the coding regions of genes are hot spots for mutation because the replication machinery is apt to slip or stutter and add or delete bases, affecting the reading frame of the coding sequence.

Gene Families

Many genes are related to other genes because of strong structural or functional similarities. These families of genes may be in close proximity on a chromosome or scattered widely throughout the genome.

The members of the **RNA gene** family do not encode for polypeptides but have RNA as their final product. Most make molecules that are involved in gene expression, such as the rRNA and tRNA families. Ribosomal RNA genes are organized in tandemly repeated clusters in a similar fashion to the different types of satellite DNA. The 18S, 5.8S, and 28S rRNA genes (or rDNA) for cytoplasmic ribosomes are located as a single transcription unit with one promoter that is tandemly repeated 30 to 40 times on each of the short arms of the acrocentric chromosomes 13, 14, 15, 21, and 22. After transcription, the RNA is processed to produce the three different rRNA sizes.

Some gene families that encode for polypeptides demonstrate very close sequence homology. The genes for the histone subunits are spread throughout the genome in multiple clusters with 61 gene copies identified and are highly conserved across species, another indication of the essential housekeeping role of histones. There is a difference of only two amino acids between cattle and garden peas of the 110 amino acids found in histone 4.

The globin gene family contains a number of subfamilies, including the myoglobin, α-globin, and β-globin subfamilies. The α-globin and β-globin gene families show a high degree of sequence similarity. The two α-globin genes are at 16p13.3 in a single cluster with one embryonic α-globin–like gene. The β-globin gene cluster is at 11p15.5 with five genes that are activated chronologically throughout the life cycle of the developing embryo, fetus, and child (Fig. 4.5). Embryonic globin synthesis (ζ-globin and ε-globin) occurs in the yolk sac in the first trimester of pregnancy but then changes to fetal liver and fetal hemoglobin (α- and γ-globin). Shortly before birth, β-globin synthesis begins, and normal adult hemoglobin takes over the oxygen-carrying role from fetal hemoglobin. Locus control regions upstream from the embryonic hemoglobin genes control expression of the genes and the correct developmental timing.

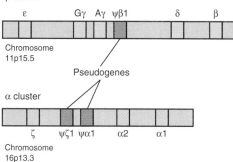

ε   Gγ Aγ ψβ1   δ   β

Chromosome
11p15.5

Pseudogenes

α cluster

ζ   ψζ1 ψα1   α2   α1

Chromosome
16p13.3

FIGURE 4.5 Both α-globin genes (α-1 and α-2) are identical and expressed in humans, which allows four alleles (two on each gene) to contribute polypeptides for incorporation as the two α-globin units needed in hemoglobin. Normal adult hemoglobin contains β-globin. If the β-globin gene is not producing a functional polypeptide, an earlier gene in the developmental progression (γ-globin) may remain active. Hemoglobin containing α- and γ-globin subunits is called fetal hemoglobin.

The various globin genes are thought to have evolved over millions of years through recombination and duplication of the genes. The two α-globin genes are identical; the two γ-globin genes in the β-globin cluster differ by only one amino acid. Within the globin gene clusters, three **pseudogenes**, which are nonfunctioning, incorrectly copied versions of the functioning genes, are also present.

The *HOX* genes are another family that occur in four separate arrangements of close clusters in four chromosomal locations. The clusters, an example of developmental genes with transcription factor function, have a great deal of similarity in organization and function. They are discussed in more detail in Chapter 10.

The immunoglobulin (Ig) gene family is a very large, highly diverse superfamily that functions within the immune system. These surface proteins all have one or more extracellular structural domains of the Ig category (Fig. 4.6) and include the immunoglobulin genes displayed on B-cell lymphocytes, the T-cell lymphocyte receptor genes, and the histocompatibility locus antigen (HLA) genes. The unique genetic structure and organiza-

tion of the Ig gene family means that a few genes allow each of the 10^{10} lymphocytes to display a unique gene product.

The immunoglobulins occur in five classes, IgM, IgG, IgA, IgD, and IgE (Fig. 4.6*B*). Each class has its own unique protein structure, but all maintain some similarity to each other. The constant region defines the class of antibody. The variable or N-terminal domains of the proteins produce the diversity of antibodies that are able to bind to a variety of antigens. The variability is created not by alternative splicing of RNA but by the random recombination of

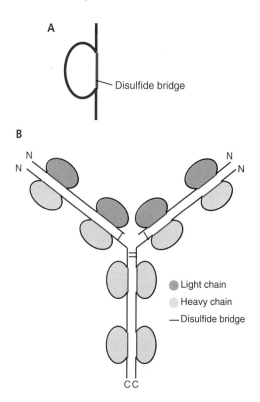

FIGURE 4.6 A. The immunoglobulin (Ig) domain consists of a series of β-pleated sheets joined by a disulfide bridge. Each member of the Ig family of genes and proteins contains at least one Ig domain in the product. **B.** A typical antibody. A typical B-cell surface immunoglobulin consists of four polypeptide chains, two heavy chains with four Ig domains each and two light chains with two Ig domains each. The heavy chains are joined together by covalent disulfide bonds. The light chains are each joined to a heavy chain by a disulfide bond. The inner or C-terminal Ig domains are constant, but the outermost or N-terminal Ig domains are variable on both heavy and light chains.

genomic DNA exons, which is perpetuated in the descendants of that particular lymphocyte. Because of lymphocyte changes, each individual is a mosaic of genomes, and even identical twins have different lymphocyte populations. The variable region of the heavy chain forms by rearrangement of individual genes from about 125 DNA segments. The process begins during B-cell development using recombinase enzymes and large-scale deletions of the sequences separating the gene segments (Fig. 4.7). A similar process occurs with light-chain genes. The recombination is purposefully imprecise; variable nucleotides are lost from the ends of the recombining gene segments and randomly chosen nucleotides are inserted, greatly increasing the diversity of the variable regions.

Mitochondrial Genome

Mitochondria, the energy producers of the cell, contain their own circular DNA and reproduce by dividing in two. Each mitochondrion contains 5 to 10 copies of 6-kb-long DNA, and each copy encodes 37 genes, including 2 rRNAs, 22 tRNAs, and 13 subunits of the oxidative phosphorylation system within the mitochondria. The mitochondrial triplet code differs slightly from the nuclear triplet code. Many more proteins are used within the mitochondria but are encoded by nuclear DNA and the products transported into the mitochondria. Mitochondrial DNA is more typical of prokaryotic DNA; it lacks introns and nucleosomes and has a circular form. Mutations occur at a much greater rate than in nuclear DNA.

Mitochondria do not have a mitotic spindle apparatus; thus, the replicated circular DNA segregates randomly as splitting of the mitochondrion occurs. The many mitochondria within the cytoplasm of a cell segregate randomly to the prospective daughter cells.

EPIGENETICS

Gene structure and organization are further influenced by control mechanisms that cause DNA to be modified or influenced without altering the inherited DNA sequence and that may even be inherited in a stable fashion. This

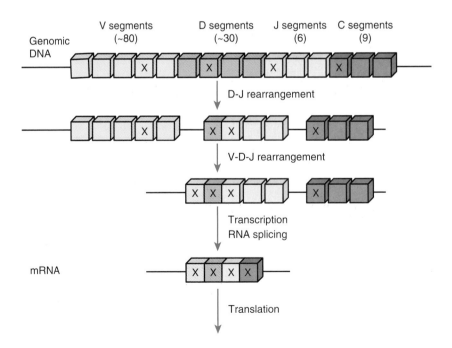

FIGURE 4.7 Rearrangement of the heavy chain genome in a B-cell lymphocyte to generate antigen specificity and the class of immunoglobulin. After the randomly selected segments are joined, the VDJ unit behaves as the single first exon. The C segments provide the remainder of the exons. V, variable; D, diversity; J, joining; C, constant.

form of regulation, an important aspect of interaction with the genome, has been termed **epigenetics**. Epigenetic modification occurs normally within cells, with transcriptional control of developmental genes and tissue-specific genes, inactivation of the X chromosome in females, gene silencing as part of aging, and inactivation of some genes that are differentiated by the parent of origin.

Methylation

Cytosine nucleotides on the 5′ side of a guanine nucleotide (CpG) are prone to methylation at the 5 position by cytosine methyltransferase (Fig 4.8). The resulting 5-methylcytosine is unstable and prone to deamination and conversion into thymine. Although the number of CpG dinucleotides has decreased over the course of evolution because of the conversion to a thymine nucleotide, the CpG density has not decreased in certain areas of DNA. These **CpG islands** often mark the 5′ ends of genes, particularly in housekeeping or developmental genes and some tissue-specific genes, and they may be found near the promoter.

Methylation of CpG islands near the promoter of a region initiates a process that silences the expression of the gene. Methylated CpGs are targets for binding by proteins such as methylated CpG-binding protein 2 (MeCP2). MeCP2 is essential as a repressor of transcription and timing of embryonic development. Once bound to the methylated CpG, MeCP2 recruits histone deacetylase (HDAC). The removal of acetyl groups from the histone tails permits condensation of the chromatin and inactivation of transcription.

Rett syndrome, a neurodevelopmental disorder of early postnatal brain growth, is caused by a dominant mutation of the MeCP2 gene at Xq28 in 80 to 85% of affected girls. Rett syndrome occurs almost exclusively in girls and has an incidence of about 1 in 10,000 births. The syndrome is usually sporadic and rarely familial. Disease onset is in early childhood. Clinical features include mental retardation, behavioral changes, movement disturbances, loss of speech and hand skills, ataxia, apraxia, irregular breathing with hyperventilation while awake, and frequent seizures. Its classical feature is wringing of the hands in front of the face, with the girl paying complete attention to the motion and unable to attend to anything else. Although Rett syndrome is the first disorder to be associated with abnormal transcription repression, it is not yet known how the clinical phenotype results from the mutation.

X Inactivation

Genes may be inactivated over broad regions of a chromosome or over an entire chromosome. In any individual with more than one X chromosome (e.g., 46,XX; 47,XXY), an entire X chromosome is inactivated in each cell. The **X inactivation** begins shortly after fertilization and is entirely random. Once it is determined which X is to be inactivated, that same X is inactivated in all progeny of that cell. As a result, males and females have the same quantity of proteins formed from genes on the X chromosome, even though females have two X chromosomes. Because females have two different cell lines due to the random inactivation of one of the X chromosomes, all females are mosaic with respect to the expression of their X-linked genes. If a woman has an abnormal gene on one of her X chromosomes, she may exhibit some symptoms depending on the tissue distribution of the cells expressing that particular X chromosome.

Mechanism

The actual mechanism of X inactivation is just beginning to be understood. It does not result in complete inactivation of the X chromosome; approximately 15% of the genes continue to be expressed. An X inactivation center at Xq13 is always present in cells, even

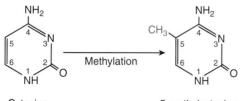

Cytosine   5-methylcytosine

FIGURE 4.8 CpG dinucleotides are a target for methylation.

in those with a structurally abnormal X chromosome. The *XIST* gene (X inactivation—specific transcript) in this inactivation center produces a noncoding RNA, which coats the DNA of the X chromosome (Fig. 4.9). Shortly after the RNA coating occurs, methylation of the lysine in the tail of histone 3 takes place and initiates chromatin condensation and conversion into facultative heterochromatin. The mechanism of propagation of inactivation along the length of the chromosome is not well understood, but it is thought that long repeat sequences interspersed in the genome facilitate inactivation. The condensed X chromosome may be observed under the microscope as a **Barr body** at the periphery of the nucleus in some 46,XX cells.

The X chromosome control element (Xce) occurs in mice, and its existence is hypothesized in humans. The Xce is located toward the Xq telomere and affects which X is selected for inactivation. Chromosomes with a strong *Xce* allele are more likely to remain active, whereas those with a weak *Xce* allele are more likely to be inactive.

Significance

X inactivation patterns assume clinical significance in the presence of a structurally abnormal X chromosome and changes in X-linked genes associated with a severe phenotype. Unbalanced structural abnormalities of the X

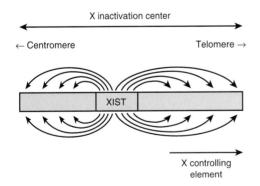

FIGURE 4.9 There appears to be an X controlling element that influences the "random" inactivation and relative proportion of inactivation of the X chromosomes. *XIST* (X inactivation specific transcript) encodes a noncoding RNA, which coats the *cis*-X chromosome and appears to remain associated with it.

chromosome (deletions and duplications) result in preferential inactivation of the structurally abnormal X chromosome, which limits the effect of the structural abnormality on an individual. However, if the individual also carries a mutation in an X-linked gene found on the structurally normal X chromosome, the mutated gene is now active in most cells because of the nonrandom inactivation pattern. Nonrandom inactivation is also seen in translocations involving the X chromosome and an autosome. In the balanced carrier (one normal autosome, one derivative autosome with X fragment, one normal X chromosome, one derivative X chromosome with autosome fragment), the normal X chromosome is preferentially inactivated. Inactivation of the derivative X chromosome results in loss of function of the autosomal fragment or a partially monosomic phenotype for the autosome. Monosomic phenotypes are highly deleterious and frequently incompatible with survival. In the unbalanced version of an X autosomal translocation (two normal autosomes, one normal X chromosome, one derivative X chromosome with autosome fragment), the derivative X chromosome is preferentially inactivated, which results in minimization of the phenotype through inactivation of the partially trisomic autosomal state.

Nonrandom X inactivation patterns are also associated with selective female survival in X-linked disorders, which are lethal in males or less severe in females carrying X-linked mutations. (A critical thinking exercise involving incontinentia pigmenti is included in the Web-based teaching resources.)

Even random X inactivation may alter expression of X-linked disorders in women. Duchenne muscular dystrophy is an X-linked disorder caused by mutations in the dystrophin gene at Xp21.2 associated with progressive myofiber degeneration of striated skeletal and cardiac muscle. The disorder affects males. Onset is in early childhood, and it usually results in death by late adolescence or early adulthood. Because of the muscle degeneration, the muscle enzyme creatine kinase is released into the bloodstream; this results in more than 10 times the normal amount of enzyme. Women who carry the abnormal dystrophin gene do not have muscle weakness or decreased life expectancy, but approximately 50% have a creatine kinase level of 2 to 10 times normal. Other women with known mutations in the dystrophin gene have a completely normal creatine kinase level. Although women with high levels of creatine kinase are likely to be carriers, women with normal levels may also be carriers. Serum levels of creatine kinase cannot be used to determine carrier status in women.

Factor VIII deficiency (hemophilia A) is another X-linked disorder in which X activation may play a role. In hemophilia A, men have a significant deficiency in blood clotting and may have debilitating or life-threatening bleeding after relatively minor trauma. Only about 10% of women who carry the mutation in the factor VIII gene have abnormally low factor VIII clotting activity. In addition, factor VIII clotting activity in plasma is increased with pregnancy, oral contraceptive use, aerobic exercise, and chronic inflammation. Furthermore, factor VIII clotting activity is approximately 25% lower in individuals in blood group O than in those in other blood groups. The presence of factor VIII clotting activity is an unreliable method of detecting carriers of hemophilia A because of this combination of X inactivation and environmental effects.

Parent-of-Origin Effects: Genetic Imprinting

Another type of epigenetic control is the normal inactivation of genes by CpG methylation based solely on the parental origin of the gene (**imprinting**). (Note that *genetic imprinting* should not be confused with *psychological imprinting*.) Only 60 to 100 genes demonstrate control of gene expression according to the parent of origin. In these gene pairs, expression of a single allele is the normal state. The gene that is not expressed or silent is imprinted (Fig. 4.10); silencing occurs through methylation of CpG islands. Gene pairs which are controlled in this fashion tend to be located in clusters with other imprintable genes and may be controlled by a common mechanism.

Typical situation in most genes

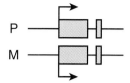

Maternal expression; paternal imprint

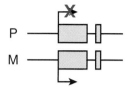

Paternal expression; maternal imprint

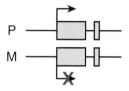

FIGURE 4.10 An imprinted gene is an unexpressed gene. An allele that is normally inactivated when inherited from the father is a paternally imprinted gene. An allele that is normally inactivated when inherited from the mother is a maternally imprinted gene. P, allele inherited from the paternal side; M, allele inherited from the maternal side.

They are significantly involved in growth control and neurobehavior. Some genes may be imprinted only in specific tissues. The unique aspect of imprinting is that the same pattern of expression is not only transmitted to daughter cells but also to subsequent generations in accordance with the parent transmitting the allele to the child. Some genes always exhibit maternal imprinting, in which the allele inherited from the mother is inactivated; some exhibit paternal imprinting, in which the allele inherited from the father is inactivated. A maternally imprinted inactivated allele inherited from a man's mother will be the active allele when the man passes that allele to his child. Another genetic allele may be paternally imprinted and inactivated in the same man because he inherited it from his father; the allele will remain inactive when the man passes that allele to his child. The mechanism for the resetting is unknown.

Diseases may occur when the imprinting mechanism does not function properly, the normally active gene carries a mutation, or both copies of a chromosomal region are inherited from the same parent. Examples of classic human disorders associated with imprinting are Beckwith-Wiedemann syndrome (chromosome 11), Prader-Willi and Angelman syndromes (chromosome 15), Russell-Silver syndrome (chromosome 7), and Albright hereditary osteodystrophy (chromosome 20). A few examples are discussed in detail later.

Uniparental Disomy

Uniparental disomy (UPD), which occurs when both copies of the same chromosome or chromosomal region are inherited from the same parent, is capable of disrupting genetic control mechanisms. UPD has no demonstrable effect in many regions of the genome but may produce an abnormal phenotype if it occurs in regions containing imprinted genes; this is due to disruption of the balance between maternally and paternally inherited alleles. UPD of the entire genome may occur in some human conceptions and have profound effects upon the phenotype because of the disruption of many imprinted genes. Diploid conceptions containing all paternal contributions develop as hydatidiform moles of the placenta with a lack of embryonic structures (Fig. 4.11). Diploid conceptions containing all maternal contributions develop into ovarian teratomas or dermoids consisting of disorganized but well-differentiated collections of adult tissues (hair, bone, teeth, and skin) without any placental structures. Triploid conceptions show a phenotypic difference depending on the diandric or digynic status of the fetus. Diandric fetuses are smaller and have a partially hydatidiform placenta. UPD of a single chromosomal region may result in disruption of the normal imprinting pattern in the region and result in an abnormal phenotype.

Disorders Caused by Disruptions of Parent-of-Origin Effects

Disorders caused by disruptions of parent-of-origin effects due to changes in genomic imprinting regions are extremely complex, with complicated inheritance patterns. Regions may be altered by small mutations in imprinting control elements, changes in epigenetic modifications, deletions or duplications of chromosomal segments, and uniparental disomy of parts of chromosomes or entire chromosomes. Active investigations constantly produce new information.

Beckwith-Wiedemann syndrome is characterized by somatic overgrowth, resulting in large-for-gestational-age infants, enlarged organs (e.g., kidney, liver, pancreas, tongue), umbilical hernia, neonatal hyperinsulinemia, and a predisposition to pediatric embryonal tumors (Fig. 4.12). The syndrome is associated with genetic or epigenetic abnormalities in a cluster of imprinted genes found within a genomic region of approximately 1 Mb on chromosome 11p15, where genes are expressed from either the paternal or maternal

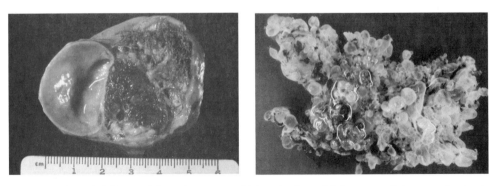

FIGURE 4.11 Uniparental disomy of the entire genome. Maternal uniparental disomy results in an ovarian teratoma (**A**). Hair and skin are evident. Paternal uniparental disomy results in a hydatidiform mole (**B**). Placental structures are disorganized, and there is no fetus. (Courtesy of the Group for Research in Pathology Education, Oklahoma City, Oklahoma.)

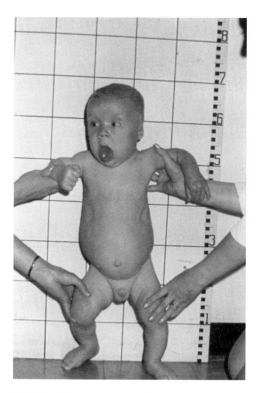

FIGURE 4.12 Infant with Beckwith Wiedemann syndrome, an example of a disorder caused by disruptions of parent-of-origin effects. Note macroglossia (enlarged tongue).

allele (Table 4.2). Approximately 50% of affected individuals have a defect in Beckwith-Wiedemann syndrome imprinting center 2, resulting in abnormal methylation of *KCNQ1OT1*. Approximately 20% of affected individuals have uniparental disomy of the genomic region, resulting in abnormal methylation of *KCNQ1OT1* and *H19*. If *KCNQ1OT1* is the only location of abnormal methylation, the individuals do not develop any pediatric tumors.

Prader-Willi syndrome and **Angelman syndrome** involve the 15q11–q13 region. Both syndromes were originally localized to this well-studied region because of a cytogenetically observed deletion. Prader-Willi syndrome is characterized by genital hypoplasia, neonatal hypotonia, associated feeding difficulty progressing to excessive eating and obesity, short stature, and small hands and feet. It occurs when genes that are normally expressed by the paternal allele are absent or inappropriately imprinted. In 70% of cases, there is a deletion of the paternal copy of 15q12; in 25% of cases, there is an associated UPD of the maternal chromosome; and in 5% of cases, there is association with disruptions of the maternal

TABLE 4.2 GENES LOCATED IN 11p15.5 REGION

GENE	ENCODES	EXPRESSION
IGF2	Insulin-like growth factor 2 or somatomedin A	Paternal expression; loss of imprinting in Beckwith-Wiedemann syndrome
H19	Noncoding RNA	Maternal expression in adult skeletal and cardiac muscle; shares enhancer with *IGF2*
INS	Insulin	Biallelic expression in tissues
KCNQ1	Potassium channel, voltage gated	Biallelic expression; mutated in long QT syndrome
KCNQ1OT1 (*KCNQ1* overlapping transcript 1)	Noncoding RNA within intron 10 of *KCNQ1*	Paternal expression; loss of imprinting in Beckwith-Wiedemann syndrome
BWSIC1 *BWSIC2* *BWSIC3*	Beckwith-Wiedemann syndrome imprinting centers 1,2,3	Disruptions associated with Beckwith-Wiedemann syndrome
CDKN1C	Cyclin-dependent kinase inhibitor 1C	Maternal expression

imprinting control element. Angelman syndrome is characterized by mental retardation, microcephaly, ataxic gait, inappropriate laughter, and seizures. Angelman syndrome occurs when genes that are normally expressed by the maternal allele are absent, disrupted, or inappropriately imprinted. In 70% of cases, there is a deletion of the maternal copy of 15q12; in 20% of cases, there are mutations in the *UBE3A* (ubiquitin protein ligase 3) gene; in 5% of cases, there is paternal UPD; and in 5% of cases, there are disruptions of the paternal imprinting control element.

An additional concern has arisen with the observation of an increased incidence of imprinting disorders, specifically Beckwith-Wiedemann syndrome and Angelman syndrome, after the use of assisted reproduction technologies (e.g., in vitro fertilization of oocytes, intracytoplasmic sperm injection) to treat infertility. It is possible that assisted reproduction technology may alter the resetting of the imprinted alleles which normally takes place at some time in the first few cycles of cellular growth and division.

CLINICALLY RELEVANT LABORATORY TECHNIQUES

One of the first challenges in studying gene structure, organization, and control is accurate and rapid purification of the DNA to be studied. **Cloning** has been technically possible since the early 1970s; it involved propagating DNA fragments for several days inside foreign hosts such as viruses, bacteria, and yeast cells. Cloning, which implies that all descendants of the original fragment of DNA are identical to the original, is necessary to amplify the original quantity of DNA to provide unlimited material for experimental study.

Polymerase Chain Reaction

Since the mid-1980s, **polymerase chain reaction** (**PCR**) has been available and has revolutionized molecular genetics by permitting rapid amplification of DNA, allowing rapid analysis. PCR can amplify a desired DNA sequence hundreds of millions of times in a matter of hours. Rapid and easy to perform, the process is highly specific, automated, and capable of amplifying minute amounts of DNA, even DNA from badly degraded cells that would be difficult to isolate using other techniques. For these reasons, PCR has had a major impact on clinical medicine, genetic disease diagnostics, and forensic science.

For amplification of a segment of DNA using PCR, the sample is first heated so that the DNA separates into two single strands. It is cooled slightly, and a heat-stable DNA polymerase is used to synthesize new strands. This process results in duplication of the original DNA; each of the new molecules contains one original strand of DNA and one new strand of DNA. Then each of these strands is used to create two new copies. The cycle of separating and synthesizing new DNA is repeated as many as 30 or 40 times, leading to more than one billion exact copies of the original DNA segment. PCR is automated; a thermocycler is programmed to alter the temperature of the reaction every few minutes. The entire cycling process can be completed in just a few hours.

Basic PCR may start with a sample of genomic DNA. To amplify a specific target DNA coding sequence, mRNA produced by the DNA may be isolated and converted to DNA using reverse transcriptase (RT); the resulting complementary DNA (cDNA) consists solely of the transcribed regions of DNA. Amplification of the cDNA is known as RT-PCR. Some knowledge of the target DNA sequence is required to design primers that are specific for sequences flanking the target. It is important to avoid repetitive sequences as primers to permit amplification of the single targeted sequence. A quantitative type of PCR simultaneously amplifies and measures the concentrations of the target sequences; this process is known as real-time PCR. It is used to quantify gene expression and to screen for mutations and SNPs.

Sequencing

DNA sequencing is used to determine the normal sequence of genes and for detection of mutations within genes. Prior to the Human Genome Project, sequencing was done manually using gel electrophoresis. One of the major contributions of the Human Genome Project has been the development of technology that rapidly assesses and analyzes genes. Current methods involve the synthesis of DNA in four reactions using one of the deoxynucleotides and a small portion of corresponding dideoxynucleotides that serve to block synthesis and terminate the chain at random positions (Fig. 4.13). A different-colored fluorescent label is used in each reaction. Electrophoresis of the combined reactions uses a long thin capillary tube filled with gel. The shorter segments migrate faster through the gel, and a monitor detects the different fluorescent labels in order as they progress through the gel. The computer compiles a graphic representation of the sequence (Fig. 4.14). View the sequencing education kit from the Human Genome Project referenced at the end of the chapter for further information.

Sequencing is the most sensitive method for detection of mutations. It is usually targeted to coding regions, however, and is less likely to detect promoter or intron changes. The computer does not detect deletions or duplications of large regions of the gene; it reads one base in the sequence region in the same way that it would interpret two homozygous bases. It also does not distinguish between single-nucleotide polymorphisms that do not affect the phenotype and missense mutations that have an effect.

Denaturing High-Performance Liquid Chromatography

Technology continues to advance to permit increased efficiency in screening the genome. **Denaturing high-performance liquid chromatography** (DHPLC) is a large-scale chromatographic method used to detect sequence polymorphisms and small deletions or insertions. A combination of normal and mutated DNA can undergo strand separation by heating and rejoining through cooling. The random rejoining causes some mismatching, with a bubble in the DNA helix due to the mis-

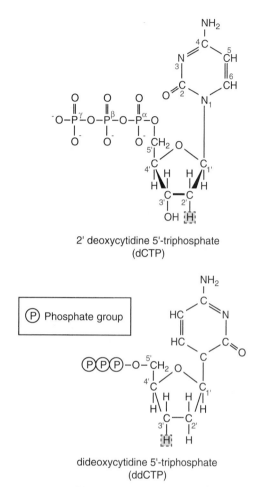

2' deoxycytidine 5'-triphosphate
(dCTP)

P Phosphate group

dideoxycytidine 5'-triphosphate
(ddCTP)

FIGURE 4.13 DNA sequencing reagents. The normal deoxynucleotide has a hydroxy group at the 3' position of the deoxyribose ring. This position normally bonds with the next nucleotide in the chain. In dideoxynucleotides, a hydrogen in the 3' place blocks additional synthesis.

match (**heteroduplex**) (Fig. 4.15). Changes in DNA methylation status at defined loci can also be assessed with DHPLC-based methodologies and used to obtain information on gene expression.

Microarray Analysis

DNA **microarray**, one of the major advances in functional genomics, offers a set of analyses that provide rapid substantial information at the DNA, RNA, or protein

MLH1 control

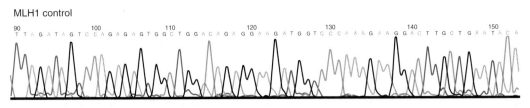

FIGURE 4.14 Results of automated sequencing. Each base is marked by a different color. Both alleles of a gene are usually included in the target DNA and are sequenced simultaneously. As long as the sequence is identical, only one curve is seen in each location (homozygosity). A single nucleotide polymorphism or a missense mutation in one allele would appear as two curves in one position. A frameshift mutation would disrupt the curves for the remainder of the sequence.

level. Its ability to study expression of several thousand genes in the genome in a single experiment is revolutionary (Fig. 4.16). It permits the rapid and efficient simultaneous analysis of thousands of nucleic acid hybridization experiments using microelectronic fabrication, miniaturization, and integration with bioinformatics.

The use of microarray, or chip, analysis has begun to alter treatment options in cancer and transplantation medicine by identifying genetic changes and cellular phenotypes that are not distinguishable by conventional microscopic analysis. The first correlation of gene expression with disease outcome was published in 2000. Diffuse large B-cell lymphoma had been marked by a 60% mortality rate and lack of response to therapy. Gene expression microarray showed two distinct sub-

populations of the lymphoma that were not detectable by conventional histology. The difference in therapeutic response correlated directly with the difference in gene expression.

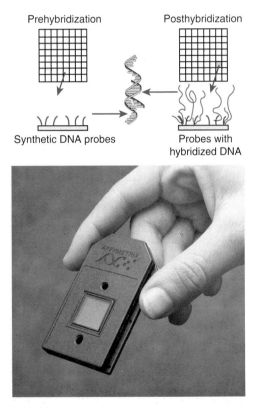

FIGURE 4.16 DNA microarray, or chip, technology entails placement of thousands of synthetic DNA probes on microchips. The DNA to be analyzed is hybridized with the probes on the chip, and the computer interprets the results, producing an analysis of the varying degrees of hybridization. Inset: GeneChip probe array. (Photo reprinted with permission from Affymetrix, Santa Clara, California.)

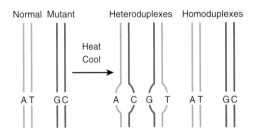

FIGURE 4.15 Denaturing high-performance liquid chromatography. Normal DNA segments are combined with a similar segment to be tested. The DNA strands are separated by heating and allowed to rejoin randomly. Any small mismatches in sequence result in a bubble in the helix or a heteroduplex. The heteroduplexes can easily be separated by chromatography.

ETHICS   DNA Profiling and its Uses

DNA fingerprinting has revolutionized forensics. This technique permits accurate identification of victims of disasters and armed conflicts, suspects of rape and violent crimes, and fathers in unresolved paternity issues. Until the mid-1980s, physical fingerprinting was considered the forensic evidence of choice. Since then, DNA analysis has become the clearest way to identify a single individual.

In 1990, the Federal Bureau of Investigation (FBI) established the Combined DNA Index System (CODIS) as a DNA profile repository for convicted offenders. International law enforcement agencies, such as Interpol, also support an international DNA profile database. The DNA Identification Act of 1994 formalized the FBI's authority to establish a national DNA index for law enforcement purposes. As of November 2004, all 50 states participate in CODIS. Law enforcement agencies can use CODIS to search the database for possible DNA matches with known convicted offenders, or they can search to link evidence from a seemingly unrelated crime with one that may have been committed by the same unidentified offender. To protect the civil rights of individual offenders, certain information is excluded from the database, such as names or data regarding physical traits, predisposition to disease, or criminal record. Search requests may be made only for the investigation or prosecution of an offense or as otherwise authorized by a court.

The national legislation permitting CODIS is limited to DNA profiles only from convicted offenders. However, many states allow the entry of profiles into their own local systems of individuals only suspected of committing crimes. Consider the following questions:
- How large should the database be?
- Does the benefit of protection of society through reliable suspect identification outweigh the infringement on personal freedom and the risk of government excess?
- To what degree should the database be expanded?
- Should samples continue to be limited to convicted offenders or be extended to arrested individuals or those under suspicion for a crime?
- Would you be willing to have your DNA profile placed in a national database?

USMLE-Style Questions

1. All individuals with more than one X chromosome are mosaic at the cellular level. How does this affect individuals who carry an abnormal gene on the X chromosome?
   a. Males with Klinefelter syndrome have the same phenotype as 46,XY males.
   b. Phenotypic severity is determined by cells and tissues with the abnormal gene active.
   c. The phenotype is the same as an X-linked disorder caused by the gene.
   d. There is no effect on the individual.

The response options for items 2 and 3 are the same:
   a. Comparative genomic hybridization
   b. DNA sequencing
   c. Linkage analysis
   d. Microarray chip
   e. Polymerase chain reaction

2. What method rapidly amplifies fragments of DNA?

3. A renal transplantation patient returns for followup renal biopsy. The medical team wishes to conduct gene expression analysis of the biopsy specimen. Which process do they use?

4. Defects in type II collagen have been associated with the autosomal dominant condition known as Stickler syndrome. Associated characteristics include short stature, loose joints, cleft palate, and arthritis. Which of the following results supports the finding of a DNA polymorphism in the third codon of one *COL2A1* locus?

   a. Denaturing high-performance liquid chromatography reveals a single nucleotide difference between homologous *COL2A1* exons.

   b. FISH analysis using a *COL2A1* probe detects signals on only one chromosome 12.

   c. RT-PCR detects half of normal amounts of *COL2A1* mRNA in affected individuals.

   d. Southern blotting for intronic DNA yields normal fragment sizes.

   e. Western blotting for protein production detects no type II collagen chains.

5. A hypervariable DNA near the telomeres is a hot spot for recombination. It is useful for DNA fingerprinting. What type of DNA is it?

   a. α-Satellite DNA
   b. β-Satellite DNA
   c. Centromeric DNA
   d. Microsatellite DNA
   e. Minisatellite DNA

SUGGESTED READINGS

Alberts B, Bray D, Hopkin K, et al. Essential Cell Biology, 2nd ed. New York: Garland Science, 2004.

Alizadeh AA, Eisen MB, Davis RE, et al. Distinct types of diffuse large B-cell lymphoma identified by gene expression profiling. Nature 2000;403:503–511. *The first clinical correlation of gene expression patterns with disease outcome.*

King HC, Sinha AA. Gene expression profile analysis by DNA microarrays: promise and pitfalls. JAMA 2001;286:2280–2288.

Naber SP. Molecular pathology: diagnosis of infectious disease. N Engl J Med 1994;331:1212–1215. *Discusses the use of PCR and other molecular techniques to diagnose infectious pathogens.*

Olivieri NF. The beta-thalassemias. N Engl J Med 1999;341:99–109.

Schwartz RS. Shattuck lecture: Diversity of the immune repertoire and immunoregulation. N Engl J Med 2003;348:1017–1026.

WEB RESOURCES

http://www.genetests.org
   GeneReviews section has an excellent summary of beta-thalassemia.

http://www.ornl.gov/sci/techresources/Human_Genome/publicat/primer/prim2.html#fpcr
   Human Genome Project Information: Mapping and sequencing the human genome. Contains basic explanations of relevant laboratory techniques.

http://www.genome.gov/Pages/EducationKit/
   Human Genome Project "Exploring Our Molecular Selves" on-line education kit. Recommend downloading the "How to Sequence a Genome" kit for good visualization of the process of automated sequencing. The four most appropriate segments begin with "Sequencing reaction."

http://www.dnalc.org/resources/aboutdnafingerprinting.html
   Dolan DNA Learning Center. Cold Springs Harbor Laboratory. "DNA Fingerprinting."

http://www.fbi.gov/hq/lab/codis/index1.htm
   CODIS Combined DNA Index System. Federal Bureau of Investigation.

Changes and Repair at the Molecular DNA Level

MUTATIONS
    Types of Mutations
    Causes of Mutations
    Germline Versus Somatic Location
    Phenotypic Expression of Mutations
        Loss-of-Function Mutations
        Gain-of-Function Mutations

DNA REPAIR MECHANISMS
    Base Excision Repair
    Nucleotide Excision Repair
    Mismatch Repair
    Recombination Repair
USMLE-STYLE QUESTIONS

Medical science typically begins with a study of the normal state and progresses to a study of the abnormal state, or pathophysiology. Medical genetics and molecular medicine are no different. Understanding the normal structure of DNA and normal gene structure, organization, and control are important prerequisites to determining disease-producing or deleterious changes in the human genome.

MUTATIONS

Although changes or **mutations** in the genome occur constantly, they are limited in scope by the normal repair mechanisms within cells. If a specific change occurs commonly in the population and is not associated with a disease phenotype, it is considered a variant or **polymorphism**. Polymorphisms typically account for differences in gene expression and protein function that still allow functioning within a normal range, thus contributing to human variability. In medical genetics, harmful changes are also called mutations; mutations may be either the initial acts of change or the final results. Mutations typically refer to changes in the genome that cause sufficient change in expression or function so that a pathophysiological state results.

Changes in DNA occur at several levels. Large changes in entire DNA molecules may occur through the addition or deletion of entire chromosomes; they have been discussed as polyploidy, nondisjunction, aneuploidy, and uniparental disomy. Changes in large sections of DNA molecules may also occur through structural rearrangements of chromosomes, such as insertions, deletions, duplications, inversions, and translocations. Changes may also occur at the gene level.

Types of Mutations

Mutations may involve the change of only a single base in the DNA sequence. A single-base change that does not result in an amino acid change is a **silent mutation** (Table 5.1), which occurs because of the degeneracy of the triplet code in which more than one codon specifies any given amino acid (Table 5.2). Because of epigenetic mechanisms and protein interactions, however, a silent mutation may actually affect the genomic interaction with the other mechanisms and may subtly alter the cellular phenotype. Many single-nucleotide polymorphisms affect drug metabolism and other events. This is discussed in more detail in Chapter 11.

A single-base change that results in a changed amino acid is a **missense mutation**. Some missense mutations cause abnormal phenotypes, and others cause amino acid polymorphisms with no clinical consequences. It is frequently not possible to predict the phenotype from the sequence information alone, and protein function must be assessed or the change

TABLE 5.1 EXAMPLES OF MUTATION NOTATION

NOTATION	TYPE OF MUTATION	MOLECULAR CHANGE	PHENOTYPIC CHANGE
810G>A (A270A)[a]	Silent	Guanine changed to adenine at base 810 with no effect on alanine at codon 270	None
1346A>G (Y431C)	Missense	Adenine changed to guanine at base 1346, changing tyrosine to cysteine at codon 431	Unknown without study of protein function
961A>T (K303X)	Nonsense	Adenine changed to thymine at base 961 changing lysine to stop at codon 303	Deleterious
187delAG	Frameshift	Adenine and guanine deleted at base 187	Deleterious
insC974	Frameshift	Cytosine inserted at base 974	Deleterious
387delC (N129fsX208	Frameshift	Cytosine deleted at base 387, changing amino acid sequence after asparagine at codon 129, terminating in stop at codon 208	Deleterious

[a]Mutations may be designated either by the change in the DNA sequence or by the change in the amino acid sequence. DNA sequence changes only are used for frameshift and intronic mutations.

linked to disease in multiple individuals in the population. A missense mutation that results in a change in the amino acid category (acidic to basic, polar to nonpolar) may be more likely to be deleterious. Until proven otherwise, a missense mutation may be referred to as a "variant of uncertain significance."

A single-base change that changes an amino acid to a stop codon is a **nonsense mutation**. These invariably result in premature truncation of the protein product and are considered deleterious.

The insertion or deletion of bases in anything other than a multiple of three disrupts the reading frame of the genetic code, resulting in creation of a new stop codon within several codons or an unstable protein, which is degraded by the cell. This is a **frameshift mutation** and is always considered deleterious. The insertion or deletion of bases in a multiple of three must be evaluated in the same way as a missense mutation with assessment of protein function or linkage to affected individuals in the population.

Mutations may also alter the recognition sequences needed for accurate splicing of introns. The 3′ end of an exon ends in AG, and the 5′ adjacent intron begins with a GT (**splice donor**). The 3′ end of the intron ends in AG (**splice acceptor**). A change in any of these sequences may result in abnormal removal of the intron. A mutation at the end of an exon may be classified as a silent mutation because of its lack of effect on amino acid sequence yet may produce an abnormal phenotype because it alters the exon splice junction sequence. For example, the last four bases of an exon are UUAG, and the first two bases of the next exon are AA. The reading frame for this particular gene is split between

TABLE 5.2 TRANSLATION OF mRNA TO AMINO ACID SEQUENCE

1ST BASE 2ND BASE		U			C			A			G		
U	UUU	Phe	F	CUU	Leu	L	AUU	Ile	I	GUU	Val	V
	UUC			CUC			AUC			GUC		
	UUA	Leu	L	CUA			AUA	Met	M	GUA		
	UUG			CUG			AUG			GUG		
C	UCU	Ser	S	CCU	Pro	P	ACU	Thr	T	GCU	Ala	A
	UCC			CCC			ACC			GCC		
	UCA			CCA			ACA			GCA		
	UCG			CCG			ACG			GCG		
A	UAU	Tyr	Y	CAU	His	H	AAU	Asn	N	GAU	Asp	D
	UAC			CAC			AAC			GAC		
	UAA	STOP	X	CAA	Gln	Q	AAA	Lys	K	GAA	Glu	E
	UAG	STOP	X	CAG			AAG			GAG		
G	UGU	Cys	C	CGU	Arg	R	AGU	Ser	S	GGU	Gly	G
	UGC			CGC			AGC			GGC		
	UGA	STOP	X	CGA			AGA	Arg	R	GGA		
	UGG	Trp	W	CGG			AGG			GGG		

Codons are always written with the 5′ nucleotide to the left. Find the first base in the codon in the first row and the second base in the codon in the first column. The third base delineates the specific amino acid or stop codon.

Alanine	A	Nonpolar
Arginine	R	Basic, positively charged polar.
Aspartic acid	D	Acidic, negatively charged polar.
Asparagine	N	Uncharged polar
Cystine	C	Nonpolar
Glutamic acid	E	Acidic, negatively charged polar.
Glutamine	Q	Uncharged polar
Glycine	G	Nonpolar
Histidine	H	Basic, positively charged polar.
Isoleucine	I	Nonpolar
Leucine	L	Nonpolar
Lysine	K	Basic, positively charged polar.
Methionine	M	Nonpolar
Phenylalanine	F	Nonpolar
Proline	P	Nonpolar
Serine	S	Uncharged polar
Threonine	T	Uncharged polar
Tryptophan	W	Nonpolar
Tyrosine	Y	Uncharged polar
Valine	V	Nonpolar

the two exons and reads UUA-GAA, encoding leucine and glutamine. A mutation changes the UUA to a UUG and preserves the leucine encoded by the original reading frame but disrupts the exon splice junction sequence. Introns are not sequenced if reverse transcriptase was used on mRNA to generate complementary DNA. Genomic DNA must be used for intron sequencing.

An example of a splice donor intron mutation is IVS5 + 13A → G, in which an adenine is changed to guanine 13 base from the 5′ end of intron 5. The splice donor and splice acceptor sites are unchanged, but the mutation creates another sequence that looks even more like a splice donor site and is used preferentially by the cell. As a result, 12 additional bases are translated before splicing occurs; the net effect is a missense mutation plus the addition of four amino acids into the reading frame of the protein. An example of a splice acceptor mutation is IVS1–1G → C, in which the first base upstream from exon 2 (the AG splice acceptor site of intron 1) is changed from a guanine to a cytosine.

Mutations in the untranslated 5′ and 3′ regions of genes or in control regions between genes may also occur. In these regions it may be very difficult to distinguish single nucleotide polymorphisms from mutations in enhancer or promoter regions. In addition, enhancer regions may be thousands of kilobases from the initiation site of the gene. Examples of mutation notation in the 5′ untranslated region are −195C → G and −13910T → C, in which the negative sign is used to indicate the number of bases upstream from the initiation of the gene.

Causes of Mutations

Mutations in DNA may occur spontaneously within the cell or in response to extraneous influences. Spontaneous changes may occur as part of DNA replication or even in the absence of replication. Chemical instability in the DNA molecule results in the regular release of purine groups from the phosphodiester chain, leaving a gap in the rungs of DNA (Fig. 5.1). Spontaneous deamination of cytosine nucleotides results in a uracil residue (Fig. 5.2) that pairs with adenine in the subsequent replication cycle, resulting in the eventual exchange of a C-G pair with a T-A pair. Spontaneous **cytosine deamination** is responsible for the formation of many single nucleotide polymorphisms from CpG dinucleotides occurring in nonregulatory regions of the genome. Intentional deamination is used in lymphocytes after rejoining of the V, D, and J portions of the immunoglobulin genes to increase the number and types of immunoglobulins produced, which further diversifies the immune response.

The normal process of cellular respiration produces wayward electrons in about 2% of

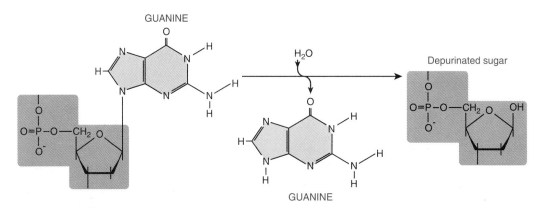

FIGURE 5.1 Depurination may release either purine base from the double-stranded DNA. The resulting mutation is repaired by recognition of the site and removal of the abnormal sugar by a special endonuclease as part of the base excision repair mechanism.

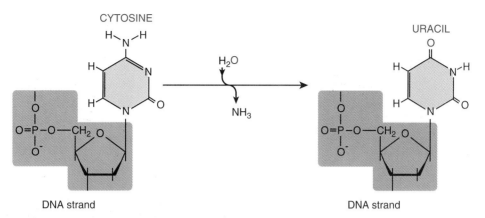

FIGURE 5.2 Deamination of the cytosine of a C-G pair results in a uracil-guanine pair. The uracil subsequently pairs with adenine in the next replication, and in the following replication the adenine pairs with thymine. After two replication cycles, the C-G pair has converted to a T-A pair in the daughter cells. Deamination mutations are repaired by the base excision mechanism.

the reactions; instead of traveling down the respiratory chain, they interact with oxygen (O_2) and create a superoxide anion (O_2^-) or another type of free radical–derived **reactive oxygen species**. The reactive oxygen species may impair lipids, proteins, and DNA. The impaired lipids may form additional reactive oxygen species (lipid peroxides) that are capable of damaging DNA by binding to deoxynucleotides. DNA damage primarily involves a preferential oxidation of guanine rings by the reactive oxygen species to form 8-oxoguanine (Fig. 5.3), which tends to pair with A rather than C. The greater the production of reactive oxygen species in the mitochondria, the lower the life expectancy of the cells and the greater the rate of aging of the organism. Overproduction of reactive oxygen species during cardiac ischemia is one of the causes of damage to the cardiac muscle. Mitochondria contain a high concentration of antioxidants to minimize damage to the cell.

Exogenous sources of mutations are common. Some wavelengths of **ultraviolet radiation** are capable of directly damaging DNA.

- Ultraviolet A (UVA) (320–400 nm). UVA, which is closest in wavelength to visible light, penetrates the ozone layer. It causes skin tanning and is necessary for vitamin D synthesis. It is also found in black lights and tanning booths. UVA does not directly damage DNA but causes increased production of reactive oxygen species, which may enhance aging of the skin and indirectly damage DNA.
- Ultraviolet B (UVB) (290–320 nm). Most UVB is blocked by the ozone layer, but the UVB that does enter the atmosphere is capable of causing cataracts and direct damage to the DNA of the skin, which may lead to skin cancer.
- Ultraviolet C (UVC) (220–290 nm). Almost all UVC is completely blocked by the ozone layer, but it is even more likely to cause DNA damage. Germicidal lamps emit bacteria-killing UVC radiation. UVB and UVC cause covalent bonds to form between adjacent thymidine bases, resulting in a cyclobutane ring or **thymidine dimer** (Fig. 5.4).

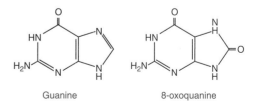

Guanine   8-oxoquanine

FIGURE 5.3 Reactive oxygen species produced in the mitochondria may oxidize guanine. The resulting 8-oxoguanine is as likely to pair with adenine as with cytosine, resulting in a mutation. Repair occurs by the base excision system.

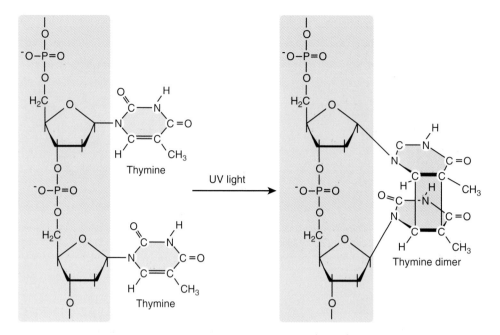

FIGURE 5.4 Thymidine dimers form in response to the energy in ultraviolet B and ultraviolet C light. Dimers are unable to participate in replication and are excised by the nucleotide excision repair pathway.

Alkylating agents and **cross-linking agents**, which may be used intentionally in cancer chemotherapy, are other exogenous sources of mutations. Alkylating agents are capable of transferring an alkyl group, usually a methyl group, onto guanine (Fig. 5.5), which distorts the DNA helix and may result in cross-linking of DNA strands through covalent joining of the resulting O^6-methyl guanine groups. The inability to separate strands during transcription and eventual replication results in cell death. Alkylating agents, which were among the first anticancer drugs, are the most commonly used chemotherapeutic agents today, with cyclophosphamide (Cytoxan) the best known example. Platinum compounds such as cisplatin are the most common cross-linking agents. Both classes are generally most useful in treating slow-growing cancers.

Aflatoxin B_1 is a toxin produced by the fungi *Aspergillus flavus* and *A. parasiticus*, mainly in tropical and subtropical countries.

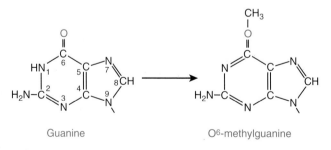

FIGURE 5.5 Alkylating agents used in cancer chemotherapy transfer an alkyl group onto guanine, promoting covalent joining of alkylated bases and preventing DNA strand replication. Repair occurs through O^6–methyl guanine–DNA methyltransferase, a specific nucleotide excision repair enzyme. Inhibition of the repair enzyme facilitates cancer chemotherapy.

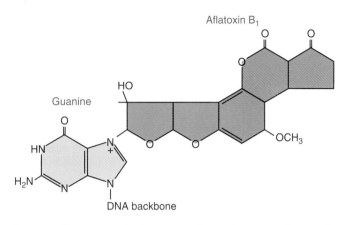

FIGURE 5.6 The entire aflatoxin B₁ molecule is covalently attached to guanine as a chemical adduct.

The toxin can be found in low levels in corn, peanuts, brazil nuts, cottonseed, and pistachios. One of the most potent mutagenic agents in nature, aflatoxin B₁ forms covalent bonds with guanine (Fig. 5.6), producing sister chromatid exchanges and chromosomal strand breaks. It is associated with an increased risk of hepatocellular carcinoma if present in significant amounts in the body. If a person has acquired the hepatitis B virus and also has significant aflatoxin levels, the risk of hepatocellular carcinoma is increased an additional 30-fold.

Polycyclic aromatic hydrocarbons found in cigarette smoke also form chemical adducts with guanine and are associated with a conversion of G to T at methylated CpG dinucleotide locations in the genome. Some genes, such as the *TP53* gene that encodes the p53 protein, are hot spots of these effects in exposed individuals. This is particularly important because p53 is normally activated in the presence of DNA damage and initiates a cascade that arrests the cell cycle in G1. If p53 cannot function correctly, damaged cells may be permitted to replicate, which increases the likelihood of cancer.

In addition to alterations in individual bases by endogenous or exogenous sources, mutations may be caused by the transcription machinery slipping either forward or backward during replication of repeated elements or misalignment during pairing of homologous chromosomes during meiosis. Slippage frequently occurs in microsatellite regions, and deletions or insertions of repeated units may occur, similar to a reader losing the way in a paragraph and skipping lines or having to reread the text several times. In cells, DNA repair mechanisms normally correct the errors, but if the errors are left unrepaired, coding or control regions may be disrupted.

Triplet repeat disorders are caused by slippage of microsatellite regions composed of trinucleotide repeat groups, primarily during meiosis. Prior to knowledge of the molecular structure, several disorders exhibited **anticipation**, in which the phenotype worsens with succeeding generations, and in some cases, the age of onset decreases. Fragile X syndrome, an X-linked mental retardation syndrome, was the first disorder found to be caused by triplet repeats. The classic features are mental retardation, large ears, prominent jaw, and macroorchidism (Fig. 5.7). When the cells of affected males were cultured under certain conditions, they were found to have a microscopically detectable fragile site at chromosome Xq28, which gave the syndrome its name. The *FMR1* gene, officially located at Xq27.3, contains a small microsatellite area of CGG repeats in the 5′ untranslated region (Fig. 5.8). Molecular analysis of this area in affected males revealed two phenomena: an enlarged and unstable CGG repeat region and methylation of the 5′ CpG island with inactivation of transcription. The CGG repeat became particularly unstable during maternal meiosis, showing a tendency

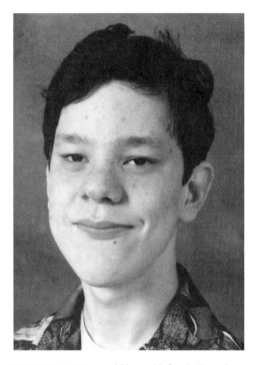

FIGURE 5.7 A 15-year-old boy with fragile X syndrome and mental retardation. Other than a prominent jaw, he has no unusual facial features.

to enlarge. Once the repeat region reached a certain size, CpG methylation occurred with subsequent gene inactivation. This provides an explanation for the inheritance pattern seen in fragile X syndrome, but it does not explain how other triplet repeat regions affect their respective genes.

Large homologous elements that are present in tandem on the chromosome are prone to **unequal crossing over** during meiosis.

This contributes to duplication of gene structures but may also cause deletion of a chromosomal region. The genes for the red and green cone pigments are on chromosome Xq28. Both red and green cone pigments differ from each other only by 15 amino acids. The red and green cone pigment genes each have six exons, and even the introns are extremely similar. They are arrayed as a single red pigment gene followed by one or more green pigment genes (Fig. 5.9A). The high degree of homology predisposes the genes to unequal crossing over, resulting in deletion or duplication of entire genes (Fig. 5.9B) or in the formation of hybrid forms (Fig. 5.9C) (Box 5.1).

Germline Versus Somatic Location

For most deleterious mutations in a coding region of the genome, the result is death of that single cell and not overall harm to the person. Some mutations, however, alter the cellular phenotype but allow continued cellular replication. These mutations may produce an abnormal phenotype in the daughter cells and may be responsible for the development of disease over time (see Chapter 8). If the new mutation occurs in the non—gamete-forming cells of the body (**somatic cells**), the consequences of the changes are limited to the person in whom the changes occurred. If the new mutation occurs in the cells that ultimately form the gametes (**germline cells**), the change may be transmitted to subsequent generations.

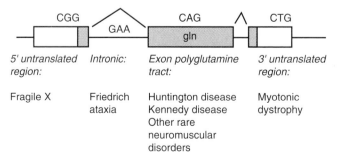

FIGURE 5.8 Classes of triplet repeat mutations. Triplet repeat regions have been found in all locations of the gene. Those that form polyglutamine tracts in the coding region tend to require fewer numbers of repeats to cause an abnormal phenotype.

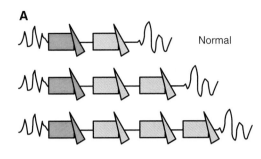

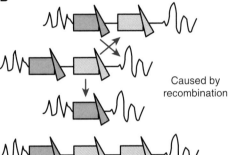

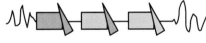

FIGURE 5.9 A. Red-green gene arrays. A red pigment gene (*gray*) is followed by one or more green cone pigment genes (*blue*). Only the first two genes in the array are expressed. **B.** Unequal pairing of nearly identical regions during meiosis results in loss of green cone pigment genes (*blue*) on some chromosomes and duplication on others. **C.** Generation of red–green hybrid genes. Unequal pairing may yield hybrid gene forms, causing altered color perception.

Phenotypic Expression of Mutations

Knowledge of the genotype—the exact change in either DNA or amino acid sequence—is important, but knowledge of the phenotype, the effect on the function of either the cell or the organism, is even more so because of the po-

tential for observable changes which may be deleterious or beneficial.

Loss-of-Function Mutations

Loss-of-function (LOF) mutations produce either a reduced amount or a reduced activity of the product. LOF mutations have minimal

BOX 5.1

Color Vision

Color disturbances are more likely to occur in males, because only one X chromosome is present, and 8% of males have some form of red-green color blindness. Absence of green pigment genes (deuteranopia), absence of red pigment genes (protanopia), altered green absorption (deuteranomaly), and altered red absorption (protanomaly) all contribute to red-green color blindness. The majority of deficits (75%) are of the deutan variety. Blue cone monochromacy is a rare disorder with absence of both red and green function due to a deletion of the expression regulation region. Additional variation in color perception is related to a S180A polymorphism in the red pigment.

effect on the phenotype unless both alleles are affected (a **recessive** phenotype). If no product or function results from an allele, it is a **null allele**. A single null allele may result in 50% reduction in product level. In many cases, this level is sufficient for normal function in the heterozygote, and two null alleles would be needed for an abnormal phenotype, resulting in the "recessive" designation. In a few circumstances, **haploinsufficiency** occurs; a 50% product level results in an altered phenotype, which appears to be caused by a mutation in only one gene (a **dominant** phenotype). In cases of haploinsufficiency, the mutations usually cause premature truncation of the protein, extreme protein instability, and no actual product within the cell.

Alagille syndrome is a dominant condition that involves the formation of decreased numbers of bile ducts within the liver, congenital heart defects, vertebral anomalies, characteristic facial features, and posterior embryotoxon of the eye (anomaly of the anterior chamber found in 8–30% of normal individuals). It is caused by mutations in the *JAG1* gene. The normal product of the gene is the jagged-1 protein, a ligand in the Notch signaling pathway that regulates cell fate and pattern formation throughout development through a process of local cell-to-cell signaling. The association of mutations in *JAG1* with Alagille syndrome indicates that Notch signaling is important in the development of the liver, heart, skeleton, facial structures, and eye. Approximately 7% of those with Alagille syndrome have a deletion of

chromosome 20p12 that completely encompasses *JAG1*. Most point mutations involve frameshift mutations with a severely truncated protein product without the transmembrane region or without the appropriate traffic signals needed for proper localization within the cell and participation in the signaling process.

Haploinsufficiency may produce changes in other signaling systems or switch mechanisms. This **dosage sensitivity** will also produce a change in phenotype in genes whose products interact with a fixed stoichiometry, such as the α-globin genes. (See Sequential Revelation Case in the Web resource for Chapter 5.)

Some heterozygous LOF mutations produce a **dominant negative** effect when the normal function of the product is lost and the abnormal product interferes with the product of the normal allele. A multimeric protein is required where the mutated product comes into physical contact with the normal product. Dominant negative mutations typically cause a more severe phenotype than does the complete absence of the product. The distinction between a dominant negative LOF mutation and a gain-of-function (GOF) mutation may be very difficult.

KCNQ1 is one of the genes in the heavily imprinted region of chromosome 11p15.5, although it is not itself imprinted (Table 4.2). It encodes the α-subunit of the slow voltage–activated potassium current (I_{Ks}), which controls duration of the action potential in the cochlea and heart. At the start of the action potential, sodium-conducting channels allow sodium to enter the cell, altering the normally negatively charged interior of the cell. The potassium channels sense the voltage change and open to allow potassium ions to flow out of the cell to restore the normal negative inside, positive outside charge. Mutations in *KCNQ1* and several other genes cause long QT syndrome, in which the QT interval of the electrocardiogram is excessively long, consistent with prolonged repolarization and a long ventricular systole. This may result in spontaneous ventricular tachycardia, resulting in syncope without warning. The tachycardia may resolve spontaneously or may deteriorate into ventricular fibrillation, which results in death unless defibrillation is performed.

Two related but separate long QT syndromes are associated with *KCNQ1* mutations. Jervell and Lange-Nielsen syndrome is characterized by severe congenital sensorineural deafness and the cardiac symptoms, and there are mutations in both alleles. Heterozygote parents have only mild cardiac symptoms. Romano-Ward syndrome, which occurs in 1 in 7000 individuals, is characterized by the cardiac symptoms only, and the symptoms in each family vary widely. The disorder is inherited in a dominant fashion, and affected individuals have a single mutated allele with 70 to 75% missense mutations. The observed mutations in Jervell and Lange-Nielsen syndrome differ from those observed in Romano-Ward syndrome. Jervell and Lange-Nielsen mutations appear to be primarily LOF mutations, whereas the Romano-Ward mutations appear to be dominant negative mutations in which the mutated allele exerts varying degrees of interference with the normal product.

Gain-of-Function Mutations

GOF mutations produce either an increased amount or increased activity of the product. GOF mutations occur when very specific changes are made to the genetic code, allowing formation of a product with enhanced activity of its existing function or a new function. As a result, the mutations are usually missense mutations that occur in a specific location in the gene or in-frame expansions of

a microsatellite repeat area, such as occurs in triplet repeat disorders.

CAG triplet expansions coding for polyglutamine tracts cause nine neurodegenerative diseases, which include Huntington disease; spinobulbar muscular atrophy; dentatorubralpallidoluysian atrophy; and spinocerebellar ataxias 1, 2, 3, 6, 7, and 17. Mouse experiments suggest that a toxic gain of function is responsible for neuronal death in most of these diseases. Proteins with an expanded polyglutamine sequence tend to form protein aggregates, which are highly toxic when directed toward the cell nucleus.

A CTG triplet repeat expansion in the 3′ untranslated region of the *DM1* gene on chromosome 19q13 causes myotonic dystrophy. The *DM1* gene codes for a serine-threonine protein kinase. Myotonic dystrophy is a multisystem disorder that affects skeletal and smooth muscle as well as other organ systems. The clinical findings are categorized into the following three phenotypes:

- Mild myotonic dystrophy (50–150 repeats) is characterized by cataract formation and mild difficulty relaxing the muscles after contraction (myotonia).
- Classic myotonic dystrophy (100–1500 repeats) is characterized by muscle weakness and wasting, myotonia, cataracts, and frequently cardiac conduction abnormalities (Fig. 5.10). It is more disabling than the mild type and may result in a shortened life span.
- Congenital myotonic dystrophy (1000 to >2000 repeats) is characterized by hypotonia and severe generalized weakness at birth and is often associated with respiratory insufficiency, mental retardation, and early death.

The scientific conundrum has been to discern how such a highly variable repeat in a transcribed yet untranslated region could account for the disease phenotype. Recent research indicates that the repeated CUG message of the translated RNA has a GOF effect in which the RNA itself has a dominant toxic effect on the cell or on transcription of other genes. A few individuals with features of

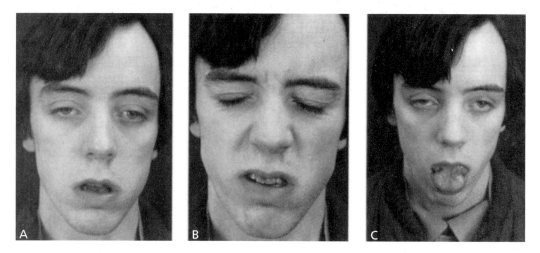

FIGURE 5.10 Patient with myotonic dystrophy. Weakness of the facial muscles causes limited facial expression and inability to open the eyes fully (**A**) and decreased ability to close the eyes tightly or generate brow furrows (**B**). Delayed relaxation of voluntary muscles after contraction appears as inability to release a hand grasp or fasciculations of the tongue (**C**) after tapping on the surface of the tongue. (Reprinted with permission from Dubowitz V. Color Atlas of Muscle Disorders in Childhood. Chicago: Year Book–Elsevier 1989:98.)

classic myotonic dystrophy have been found to have a huge expansion of CCTG (average of 5000 repeats) within intron 1 of the zinc-finger-protein 9 gene on chromosome 3q. This transcribed but untranslated mutation also has an RNA GOF effect. These findings indicate the existence of a new category of disease in which repeat expansions in RNA alter cellular function.

A few disorders with different phenotypes are now known to be caused by LOF and GOF mutations within the same gene. The *RET* gene (*re*arranged during *t*ransfection) and the *GNAS1* gene (**g**uanine **n**ucleotide-binding protein, **a**lpha-**s**timulating–activity polypeptide *1*) are the best examples to date. The *RET* proto-oncogene (defined in Chapter 8) on chromosome 10q11.2 encodes a cell surface receptor tyrosine kinase that transduces signals for cell growth and differentiation. The receptor tyrosine kinase has extracellular, transmembrane, and intracellular domains (Fig. 5.11) and functions as a dimer with another RET molecule. The extracellular domain consists of a calcium-binding cadherin-like region and a cysteine-rich region. The receptor interacts with the glial-derived neurotropic factor family of ligands. The RET tyrosine kinase in-

tracellular domain causes downstream activation of the mitogen-activated protein kinase (MAPK) signaling cascade, which alters gene transcription.

Infants with Hirschsprung disease have complete or partial intestinal obstruction due

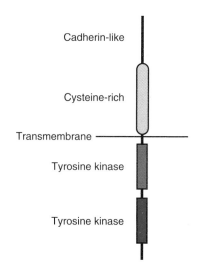

FIGURE 5.11 The RET cell surface receptor tyrosine kinase. The cadherin-like region is named for its homology to cadherin, a calcium-dependent cell adhesion protein. The cysteine-rich region forms disulfide bonds with cysteine groups in the RET dimer.

to absence of ganglion cells in a portion of the colon. Such obstruction, which may occur in 1 in 5000 newborns as an isolated finding or as part of a multisystem disease, is considered a disorder of neural crest cell migration. Isolated Hirschsprung disease has been associated with mutations in six different genes, three of which are part of the RET system. The RET receptor is normally expressed by the neural crest cells shortly after they leave the neural plate and move to colonize the entire gut. LOF mutations in the *RET* gene may be found to varying degrees in Hirschsprung disease but are present in 50% of familial cases and in as many as 70 to 80% of individuals with a long segment of the colon affected. Most mutations in the extracellular domain impair RET cell surface expression.

Multiple endocrine neoplasia type 2 (MEN2) is classified into three subtypes: MEN2A, familial medullary thyroid carcino-ma (MTC), and MEN2B (Box 5.2). All three subtypes carry a high risk of MTC. All are associated with GOF mutations in the *RET* gene. Inherited germline mutations affecting one of five cysteines in the extracellular domain (Cys609, 611, 618, 620, and 634) are responsible for the vast majority of occurrences of MEN2A and familial MTC. These mutations lead to replacement of a cysteine by another amino acid, which results in aberrant disulfide bonds and constitutive activation of the RET receptor. The mutation that causes MEN2B occurs in methionine 918 in the second tyrosine kinase domain and probably activates RET through a conformational change of the catalytic region of the receptor. LOF mutations in *RET* produce a deficiency of neural crest–derived cells, particularly in the colonic ganglions. GOF mutations in *RET* cause overproduction of neuroendocrine cells and an increase in intestinal innervation in the case of MEN2B.

G proteins, or GTP-binding proteins, are heterotrimer proteins composed of α-, β-, and γ-subunits, which transduce an extracellular signal to an intracellular second messenger pathway in either a stimulatory or inhibitory role. There are multiple family members of each type of subunit. The *GNAS1* gene encodes for a member of the α-subunit stimulatory family, which interacts with adenylyl cyclase, and ultimately cyclic adenosine monophosphate (cAMP). Many hormones function through cAMP as a second messenger.

GNAS1 has been found to have both LOF and GOF mutations. Heterozygous LOF mutations cause Albright hereditary osteodystrophy (short adult stature, obesity, brachydactyly, and ectopic ossifications), which may be associated with resistance to parathyroid hormone, thyroid-stimulating hormone, and the gonadotropins. *GNAS1* is an imprinted gene with tissue specificity. It is expressed primarily from the maternal allele in some tissues and from both alleles in most tissues. Individuals with mutations on the maternally derived allele are likely to have hormonal resistance, whereas those with mutations on the paternally derived allele do not.

BOX 5.2

Subgroups of Multiple Endocrine Neoplasia Type 2 (MEN2)

- MEN2A (90% of cases)
  - Early adulthood onset
  - MTC
  - Pheochromocytoma
  - Parathyroid adenoma or hyperplasia
- MEN2B
  - Early childhood onset
  - MTC
  - Pheochromocytoma
  - Mucosal neuromas of lips and tongue
  - Large lips
  - Ganglioneuromatosis of gastrointestinal tract
- Familial MTC
  - Middle age onset
  - MTC = medullary thyroid carcinoma.

Acquired GOF mutations in *GNAS1* lead to cellular proliferation in endocrine tissues in which cAMP is a mitogenic signal, such as growth hormone–secreting pituitary adenomas, hyperfunctioning thyroid adenomas, and Leydig cell tumors. If the same mutations occur very early in embryogenesis, they cause McCune-Albright syndrome. Individuals with McCune-Albright syndrome are mosaic for a mutation in *GNAS1* and are characterized by polyostotic fibrous dysplasia, pigment patches of the skin, and endocrinologic abnormalities, including precocious puberty, thyrotoxicosis, pituitary gigantism, and Cushing syndrome. Somatic mosaicism is the norm; thus, clinical features are highly variable from individual to individual.

DNA REPAIR MECHANISMS

DNA replication is an extremely accurate process; there is only 1 nucleotide error in every 10 million bases copied—an error rate to be envied by airline baggage handlers, the U.S. postal service, and the author and editors of this textbook. However, approximately 320 nucleotide errors occur with every cycle of cell division. The cellular DNA repair mechanisms repair most errors and increase the accuracy to 1 error in every 1 billion bases copied, which still produces 3.2 nucleotide errors with every cell division. In cultured cell lines, the cells divide a maximum number of 50 times before death. Assuming a similar limitation in living beings, 160 nucleotide errors could accumulate during the lifespan of any individual cell. Without the repair mechanisms, 16,000 nucleotide errors could result in any single cell. Several major types of DNA repair mechanisms are described in the following section.

Base Excision Repair

Base excision repair removes abnormal bases caused by DNA instability or mutagenic agents in the cell or exogenous environment. The damaged base is recognized and excised by a DNA glycosylase specific for the type of damage. The phosphoribose backbone is cut at the apurinic/apyrimidinic site

by an apurinic/apyrimidinic endonuclease, with removal of the fragment. The gap is filled by a DNA polymerase, and the final break is closed by DNA ligase. At present, no known inherited defects are associated with base excision repair. Some cancer chemotherapies generate abnormal single nucleotides, so there is interest in slowing the normal base excision repair process to augment the effects of the mutagenic treatments.

Nucleotide Excision Repair

Nucleotide excision repair deals with a large variety of DNA changes, including thymidine dimers from ultraviolet radiation and alterations by chemical adducts from environmental agents such as tobacco smoke. More than 30 proteins are involved in nucleotide excision repair in two subpathways, the ongoing process of global genomic repair and transcription-coupled repair. Nucleotide excision repair may be inactivated by four rare inherited recessive disorders—xeroderma pigmentosum (XP), Cockayne syndrome, trichothiodystrophy, and cerebro-oculo-facial-skeletal syndrome (Fig 5.12)—which are all associated with increased sensitivity to sun.

Much of the nucleotide excision repair process was discovered in the course of study-

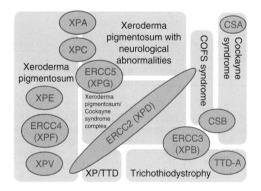

FIGURE 5.12 The clinical phenotypes (rectangles) associated with defects in nucleotide excision repair. NER genes (ellipses) superimposed on the appropriate phenotypes show the complexity of the repair system and the overlapping nature of the phenotypes. ERCC, excision repair–complementing defective, in Chinese hamster. COFS, cerebral-ocular-facial-skeletal syndrome. (Redrawn with permission from Wattendorf DJ, Kraemer KH. GeneReviews: Xeroderma Pigmentosum. www.genetests.org.)

ing XP and is named after the disease. Individuals with XP have sun sensitivity, eye involvement, and more than 1000-fold increased risk of skin and eye cancers. Acute sun sensitivity may be present from infancy, in association with severe sunburn with blistering or redness with minimal sun exposure. Pronounced facial freckling in children younger than 2 years of age is typical in XP. Affected individuals must be protected from sun and ultraviolet exposure and may develop skin cancers in sun-exposed areas at a very early age.

There are seven **complementation** groups in XP (XPA to XPG), which implies that seven different genes are involved in the production of the XP phenotype (Table 5.3). More than 90% of Japanese patients with XP have the same single-base substitution in *XPA*. Most U.S. patients have mutations in *XPC*. The children of an individual with XPA who marries an individual with XPC will have normal children, because the mutated *XPA* and *XPC* genes encode different proteins and complement each other, covering each other's functional weaknesses. XPC and other proteins bind to damaged DNA and recruit the other nucleotide excision repair factors. ERCC3 and ERCC2, components of the multimeric transcription factor that initiates transcription by RNA polymerase II, serve as helicases that unwind the DNA in opposite directions in the damaged area. XPA arrives and anchors a complex with ERCC4, which makes a single-strand nick on the 5′ side of the damage. XPA also activates ERCC5, which makes a single-strand nick on the 3′ side approximately 30 nucleotides away. DNA ligase I restores the 30-nucleotide gap.

Mismatch Repair

Mismatch repair corrects errors made during replication, which may leave a mispaired nucleotide, or mismatch. A protein complex recognizes the mismatches, excises the area on the newly synthesized strand, and resynthesizes the removed portion. At least five genes (*MLH1*, *MSH2*, *MSH6*, *PMS1*, and *PMS2*) are involved; one group of products recognizes single nucleotide mismatches, and another group recognizes loops that occur when deletions or insertions occur in microsatellite repeat areas. The genes (*Mut L* and *Mut S*) were identified initially in *Escherichia coli* and the homologs found in humans (*MLH1* is a Mut L homolog; *MSH2* is a Mut S homolog). MSH2 binds with MSH6 and is thought to slide along the DNA to single mismatches. MSH2 works with MSH3 to detect mismatch loops. Once found, MLH1 and PMS2 (single mismatches) or

TABLE 5.3 COMPLEMENTATION GROUPS OF XERODERMA PIGMENTOSA AND ASSOCIATED GENES AND PROTEINS OF THE NUCLEOTIDE EXCISION REPAIR

COMPLEMENTATION GROUP	GENE NAME	CHROMOSOMAL LOCATION	PROTEIN FUNCTION
XPA	*XPA*	9q22.3	DNA repair
XPB	*ERCC3*	2q21	TFIIH basal transcription factor complex helicase, XPB subunit
XPC	*XPC*	3p25	DNA repair
XPD	*ERCC2*	19q13.2–q13.3	TFIIH basal transcription factor complex helicase, subunit
XPE	*DDB2*	11p12–p11	DNA damage binding protein 2
XPF	*ERCC4*	16p13.3–p13.13	DNA repair
XPG	*ERCC5*	13q33	DNA repair

TFIIH, transcription factor that initiates transcription by RNA polymerase II.

PMS1 (loops) binds to the MSH2 complex and coordinates the other proteins required for excision, unwinding, and synthesis. Inherited defects in the mismatch repair system cause hereditary nonpolyposis colorectal cancer (see Chapter 8).

Recombination Repair

Recombination repair, which depends on chromosomal homology, fixes breaks in double-stranded DNA that occur during meiosis or mitosis or as a result of exposure to ionizing radiation. The *BLM* gene (see Chapter 2) works during homologous recombination to unwind the entwined chromosomes. If it is not working properly, excessive recombination occurs. An intricate network exists among DNA damage signal transducers,

cell cycle regulators, and different recombination repair processes.

In one process, the ataxia-telangiectasia mutated gene (*ATM*) encodes a protein kinase that is activated by the chromatin changes caused by ionizing radiation. The activated ATM product then phosphorylates a checkpoint kinase, which interacts further with cell cycle controllers and the *BRCA1*-associated genome surveillance complex (BASC) to initiate repairs via a mechanism that is not completely understood (Fig. 5.13). The BRCA1 and BRCA2 proteins in the BASC system interact with the Rad51 recombinase to form a nucleoprotein filament at the broken strand, facilitating repair.

Inherited mutations in the *ATM* gene cause the recessive disease ataxia-telangiectasia, which has a high degree of chromosomal insta-

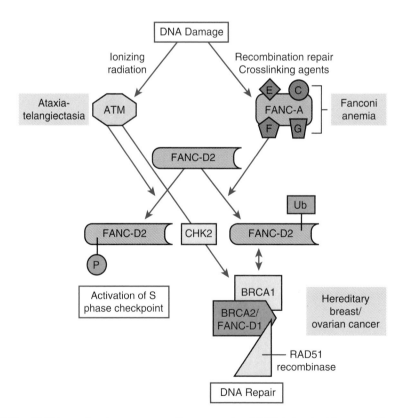

FIGURE 5.13 The *BRCA1*-associated genome surveillance complex (BASC) is involved in recognition and repair of double-stranded DNA breaks caused by ionizing radiation and repair of cross-linking agents. FANC, complementation groups associated with Fanconi anemia; ATM, ataxia-telangiectasia mutated gene; *BRCA1* and *BRCA2*, breast cancer 1 and 2 genes; CHK2, checkpoint kinase 2; Ub, ubiquitin group.

bility and cellular sensitivity to ionizing radiation. Affected individuals develop telangiectasias of the sclerae, progressive cerebellar ataxia, immune defects, and an increased likelihood of cancer. Inherited mutations in *BRCA1* or *BRCA2* cause the dominant hereditary breast/ovarian cancer syndrome, which is associated with a significant susceptibility to breast and ovarian cancer (see Chapter 8).

Another part of the BASC system responds to DNA damage and is particularly sensitive to interstrand cross-links. The genes and proteins are named after their association with Fanconi anemia, a recessive disorder that affects all bone marrow elements. Affected individuals have cardiac, renal, and limb malformations and skin hyperpigmentation, and their cells have multiple chromosomal exchanges between nonhomologous chromosomes. There are nine complementation groups in Fanconi anemia, which implies a multimeric protein or involvement in a single pathway. Not all of the *FANC* genes and products have yet been identified, but several appear to form a nuclear protein complex that interacts ultimately with BRCA1. The FANC-D1 complementation group has been shown to be the same as BRCA2.

ETHICS   Presymptomatic Testing in an Untreatable Disease

Increased understanding of the underlying molecular cause of diseases and the technical ability to perform genetic testing has meant that we can identify gene mutations in an individual and conduct tests before clinical symptoms of a disease occur. In many disorders, the presence of a mutation does not mean that development of disease is inevitable. We have learned to express caution and speak in probabilities.

Presymptomatic testing of some disorders allows preventive therapy or early detection with relatively safe treatment. Individuals in families affected by MEN2A can be tested. If a mutation is found, they can have a thyroidectomy to eliminate the risk of medullary thyroid carcinoma, which is fatal unless detected early. Individuals in families affected by long QT syndrome can be tested. If a mutation is found, they can consider having a pacemaker or implanted defibrillator to maintain normal cardiac rhythm.

In Huntington disease, however, it is believed that the presence of a mutation is almost invariably associated with the development of disease symptoms. This disorder has an average age of onset of 35 to 44 years, after many individuals have had their children. Huntington disease is caused by an expansion of a microsatellite triplet (CAG) repeat region (Fig. 5.7). Individuals with more than 42 CAG repeats develop symptoms. In the early stages, changes may be subtle; they include slight loss of coordination, small involuntary movement or twitches, difficulty in planning, and irritable or depressed mood. The movement disorder progresses, and aggressive outbursts may preclude employment. Affected individuals eventually lose the ability to move, speak, or function independently. Death usually occurs by age 55 years. There is no successful treatment or cure.

Individuals with Huntington disease can do nothing to stop the development and progression of the disease. Consequently, knowledge of mutation status prior to the development of symptoms may generate a significant sense of loss, futility, and depression, particularly if the person is already undergoing some of the psychological changes associated with Huntington disease. As a result of these concerns, scientists and families affected by Huntington disease developed a testing protocol for the presymptomatic individual that incorporates genetic counseling with psychological assessment and

(continues)

ETHICS | **Presymptomatic Testing in an Untreatable Disease** *(continued)*

counseling before the test is performed and after the results are received. Only adults are eligible to participate in presymptomatic testing.

Even with these concerns and outcomes, some individuals choose to proceed with presymptomatic mutation analysis. They receive all of the information and believe that the knowledge of their personal status is preferable to living with uncertainty. Some find that they do not have an expansion of the CAG repeat region and do not develop Huntington disease. They eventually feel a sense of relief but may have to first deal with survivor's guilt, a sense of guilt for not developing a disease that other family members may face and for whom they may become the caregiver. Some have their fears confirmed and plan with family members regarding finances and end-of-life care. A few find the news too much to handle, reject the established psychological care, and commit suicide at the first appearance of symptoms.

In a study in Britain in 2000, only 20% of those eligible for presymptomatic testing for Huntington disease chose to be tested. If you were at risk, would you have the test?

USMLE-Style Questions

1. A college student is on spring vacation in Mexico. She spends several hours on the beach without sunscreen and develops a significant sunburn. As a result, which of the following type of damage is found in her DNA?
   a. Breaks in double-stranded DNA
   b. Breaks in single-stranded DNA
   c. Purine base loss
   d. Sequence exchange of tandemly repeated DNA
   e. Thymidine dimers

2. What is the one clinical feature shared by all disorders caused by defects in DNA repair mechanisms?
   a. Autosomal recessive inheritance
   b. Increased risk of cancer
   c. Mental retardation and developmental delay
   d. Short stature
   e. Skeletal and limb abnormalities

3. A new missense mutation has been discovered in a gene. It appears to cause a very different disease from that produced by a nonsense mutation in the same region of the gene. The protein product is produced in normal quantity. A large number of unrelated individuals with this same disease have been found to have the identical missense mutation. Which of the following expressions best characterizes the mutation?
   a. Dominant negative
   b. GOF mutation
   c. Haploinsufficiency
   d. Null allele
   e. Polymorphism

4. Achondroplasia, the most common type of dwarfism, is caused by a single mutation, a G380R mutation in the transmembrane portion of fibroblast growth factor receptor 3 (FGFR3). Which of the following effects of this mutation on the gene is the most likely?
   a. GOF causing ligand-independent activation of FGFR3
   b. LOF causing reduction in extracellular affinity for fibroblast growth factor
   c. LOF causing reduced ability to activate tyrosine kinase region
   d. LOF causing reduced dimerization of receptor
   e. Recessive effect on receptor function

SUGGESTED READINGS

Vincent GM. The long-QT syndrome: bedside to bench to bedside. N Engl J Med 2003;348: 1837–1838.

Eng C. Seminars in medicine of the Beth Israel Hospital, Boston. The RET proto-oncogene in multiple endocrine neoplasia type 2 and Hirschsprung's disease. N Engl J Med 1996;335: 943–951.

Eng C, Clayton D, Schuffenecker I, et al. The relationship between specific *RET* proto-oncogene mutations and disease phenotype in multiple endocrine neoplasia type 2. International *RET* mutation consortium analysis. JAMA 1996;276: 1575–1579.

Harper PS, Lim C, Craufurd D. Ten years of presymptomatic testing for Huntington's disease: the experience of the UK Huntington's Disease Prediction Consortium. J Med Genet 2000;37: 567–571.

WEB RESOURCES

http://www.genetests.org
Reviews of Alagille syndrome, long QT syndrome, myotonic dystrophy, Hirschsprung disease, multiple endocrine neoplasia type 2, xeroderma pigmentosum, Cockayne syndrome, and hereditary nonpolyposis colorectal cancer syndrome.

http://www.ncbi.nlm.nih.gov/entrez/query.fcgi?
db=OMIM
Review of McCune-Albright syndrome, including its clinical features.

http://www.mcw.edu/cellbio/colorvision/test1.htm
Conduct your own color vision screening in this site from the Medical College of Wisconsin. See what the world looks like to someone with red-green color blindness.

http://www.hdfoundation.org/testread/hdsatest.htm
Guidelines for testing for Huntington disease (1994) from the Huntington's Disease Society of America web site of the Hereditary Disease Foundation.

Mendelian Inheritance: Observation of Phenotypes

". . .no-one can say why the same peculiarity in different individuals. . . .is sometimes inherited and sometimes not so: why the child often reverts in certain characters to its grandfather, or other much more remote ancestor; why a peculiarity is often transmitted from one sex to both sexes, or to one sex alone, more commonly but not exclusively to the like sex."

CHARLES DARWIN
On the Origin of Species by Means of Natural Selection
(1859)

The Augustinian monk Gregor Mendel (1822–1884) developed theorems that served as the foundation of medical genetics for much of the twentieth century. Beginning in 1856, he experimented with garden peas. Although he read Darwin's work with interest, he believed he had answers about the inherited characters and the patterns in which traits were transmitted from generation to generation. Mendel's work with crossing peas of different traits showed that the hybrid parent plants produced offspring showing the original traits in varying proportions, or segregation of traits. His work gave rise to the concepts of dominant and recessive traits.

Mendel's Law of Segregation states:

- Alternative versions of genes account for variations in inherited characters.

- For each character, an organism inherits two genes, one from each parent.
- If the two alleles differ, then one, the dominant allele, is fully expressed in the organism's appearance; the other, the recessive allele, has no noticeable effect on the organism's appearance.
- The two genes for each character segregate during gamete production.

Mendel's Law of Independent Assortment states that the emergence of one trait does not affect the emergence of another.

It is assumed that the reader possesses a basic knowledge of Mendelian genetics. Mendelian genetics provided many answers to the observed phenotypes of individuals with biochemical disorders or striking physical characteristics. However, in this age of molecular analysis, it is too simplistic. Mendelian genetics assumes that traits are a result of simple two-allele systems. The discussion of different mutations within the same gene in Chapter 5 demonstrates the challenges to that belief. Multiple alleles of the same gene do exist, and loss-of-function and gain-of-function mutations result in varying phenotypes. Cataloguing systems such as the Online Mendelian Inheritance in Man (OMIM) no longer categorize newly described genes as dominant or recessive but by genomic location (autosomal, X-linked, Y-linked, or mitochondrial).

Mendel did not imagine the broader spectrum of allelic possibilities, but two of his basic concepts are correct: (*a*) a gene is inherited from each parent (except for uniparental disomy), and (*b*) alleles segregate during meiosis. Mendelian genetics is so inherent in scientific thought that it is important to review it and have a good working knowledge of its applications. However, it is too simplistic in this age of molecular analysis, and its flaws at the molecular level must be recognized. Medical practitioners should be prepared for new exceptions to classic mendelian rules.

PEDIGREE CONSTRUCTION

Mendel developed his theorems on the basis of his observation of phenotypes. Human diseases are characterized by the pattern of phenotypes appearing in a family history. Therefore, all medical practitioners should be able to prepare and interpret a **pedigree**, or graphic representation of a family history. A good family medical history is one of the least expensive yet most effective tools in health care. The family history is a dynamic part of the history and should be reviewed annually and updated as necessary.

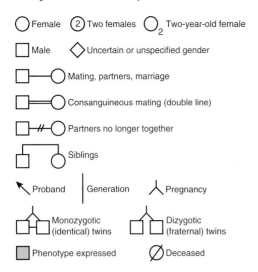

FIGURE 6.1 Commonly used symbols in pedigree construction. Family therapists use notation derived from genetic pedigree symbols but with significant differences in the structure and meaning of the lines used to join the symbols. The proband is the first affected person to be identified in a family or the person being interviewed.

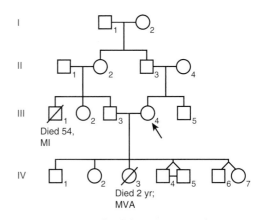

FIGURE 6.2 Sample family history using pedigree notation. MI, myocardial infarction; MVA, motor vehicle accident.

A graphic representation of pedigree construction is available on the Web site for this textbook. Figure 6.1 shows commonly used pedigree symbols. When drawing a pedigree while taking a family history, start with the proband and immediate relatives and expand downward (offspring), outward (siblings), and upward (parents and past generations). Siblings, or sibs, should be drawn in chronological order if possible. Medical history can be recorded next to the symbol (Fig. 6.2). Causes of death and ages of death should be recorded if known. Names can be recorded near symbols, or individuals can be anonymous and numbered (Fig. 6.3).

It is important to determine and record the individual's ethnicity, religious heritage, and country of origin. Many genetic disorders vary in frequency among ethnic groups. Religious heritage is important to determine whether a family has been part of a close-knit religion that may be at increased risk for genetic dis-

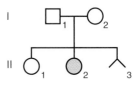

FIGURE 6.3 Specific individuals in a pedigree may be designated by a roman numeral for the generation and an arabic numeral for the position within the generation as marked sequentially from left to right. Individual II-2 has the phenotype of interest. The open wedge at II-3 indicates a pregnancy in progress. Using this notation, the proband arrow in Figure 6.2 is pointing to individual III-4.

orders, such as the Amish or the Eastern European Jews (Ashkenazi Jews).

Relatives in a family kindred are differentiated by their degree of relatedness. **First-degree** relatives (parents, siblings, children), the most closely related individuals, are shown by lines without any intervening symbols. **Second-degree** relatives (aunts, uncles, nephews, nieces, grandparents, grandchildren, half-siblings) are shown as line, symbol, line. **Third-degree** relatives (first cousins, great-grandparents) are shown as line, symbol line symbol, line. The number attributed to the degree of relatedness continues to increase as additional intervening relatives are considered. Third-degree relatives have fewer genes in common than do first-degree relatives.

Consanguinity, a blood relationship between descendants of a common ancestor, frequently occurs in some small culturally isolated populations, such as the Amish, and results in an increased number of identical genes between individuals. Consanguinity is also common in cultures with arranged marriages, such as in some Middle Eastern, Islamic, and Indian groups. Unrestricted marriage between first cousins is permitted in 19 U.S. states and the District of Columbia, but marriage between more closely related individuals is illegal in all 50 states. When taking a family medical history, the practitioner should routinely ask, "Are you (or the parents) related in any way other than through marriage?"

INHERITANCE PATTERNS

Mendelian inheritance is reserved for characteristics or disorders for which changes at a single gene locus are sufficient for the characteristic to be expressed. These changes result in inheritance patterns that can be recognized in the family history. The concept of dominant should be used if the phenotype is expressed in the heterozygous state, and the concept of recessive should be used if the phenotype is expressed only in the homozygous state. Mendelian inheritance is used only to describe the nuclear genome.

Genes themselves are not dominant or recessive. Mutations within the genes may give rise to dominant or recessive phenotypes

based on the characteristics and location of the mutations within the gene. In some cases, the phenotype observed in the family history may differ from the phenotype observed at the cellular level. For instance, individuals with an inherited susceptibility to develop cancer may appear to have a dominant phenotype in the pedigree, but a homozygous ("recessive") genetic mutation is necessary at the cellular level to allow the cancer to actually develop. (See Chapter 8 for a more detailed discussion.)

The pedigree pattern of mendelian single-gene disorders is first determined by the chromosomal location of the gene. Genes on chromosomes 1 through 22, the autosomes, are **autosomal** and have two alleles for each gene. Genes on the X chromosome are **X-linked** and have two alleles in females, one of which is on the inactivated X, and one allele in males. Genes on the Y chromosome are **Y-linked** and have only one allele. Men who are 47,XYY are always homozygous, because the Y chromosomes are identical. Once the chromosomal location is identified, phenotypes are described as **dominant** or **recessive**, and each has recognizable pedigree patterns. The distinguishing features of the varying inheritance patterns are described in the following sections.

Autosomal Dominant Inheritance (Fig. 6.4)

- Males and females are equally affected.
- Affected males and females are equally capable of transmitting the trait.
- An affected person usually has at least one affected parent.

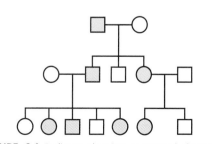

FIGURE 6.4 Pedigree showing autosomal dominant inheritance.

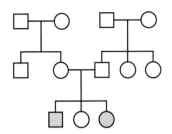

FIGURE 6.5 Pedigree showing autosomal recessive inheritance. Some texts may mark heterozygote (carrier) status, but family members rarely come to the first appointment with knowledge of carrier status.

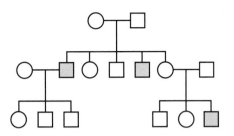

FIGURE 6.7 Pedigree showing X-linked recessive inheritance. What is the certainty of the carrier status of individuals I-2, II-6, III-1, and III-5?

X-Linked Recessive Inheritance (Fig. 6.7)

- Males are mostly affected.
- All daughters of affected males are carriers.
- Females are affected if they have a structural X cytogenetic abnormality, are 45,X, or have an affected father and a carrier mother.
- No male-to-male transmission occurs.
- Carrier females have a 50% risk of transmitting the trait to their sons and a 50% risk of transmitting carrier status to their daughters.

X-Linked Dominant Inheritance (Fig. 6.8)

- Both males and females may be affected, but more females are evident.
- Females are usually less severely affected because of random X inactivation and mosaicism.
- The pedigree may appear very similar to an autosomal dominant pedigree but without any male-to-male transmission.

- An affected person has a 50% probability of transmitting the trait to any offspring.
- The gene product is commonly a nonenzymatic protein.

Autosomal Recessive Inheritance (Fig. 6.5)

- Both parents of an affected child are usually asymptomatic carriers.
- Males and females are equally affected.
- Consanguineous partners have an increased risk of sharing the same genetic mutation and an increased risk of having affected children.
- Unaffected parents who have one affected child have a 25% risk of having an affected child with each subsequent pregnancy.
- The unaffected sibling of an affected individual has a 2 in 3 risk of being a carrier, assuming that both parents are unaffected. (Fig. 6.6).
- The gene product is commonly an enzyme.

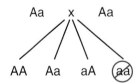

Aa   x   Aa

AA   Aa   aA   aa

FIGURE 6.6 Offspring of heterozygotes of a recessive gene. In any pregnancy, heterozygote parents have a 25% chance of having an affected homozygous child, a 50% chance of having heterozygous unaffected children, and a 25% chance of having homozygous unaffected children. If a child is known to be unaffected, the child has a 2 in 3 chance of being a heterozygote.

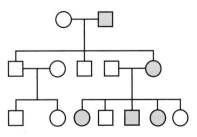

FIGURE 6.8 Pedigree showing X-linked dominant inheritance. The lack of male-to-male transmission does not prove X-linked dominant inheritance, however, because relatively few family members are shown.

Y-Linked Inheritance

- Only male-to-male transmission is observed.

GENETIC COUNSELING

In 1975, the American Society of Human Genetics defined genetic counseling as a communication process that deals with the human problems associated with the occurrence, risk of occurrence, or risk of recurrence of a genetic disorder in a family. The process helps individuals or families to do the following:

- Understand the medical facts, including the diagnosis, prognosis, and available management
- Understand the ways in which genes and other factors contribute to the disorder and the risk of occurrence in specific relatives
- Gain information about the alternatives for dealing with the possibility of recurrence
- Choose a course of action that seems appropriate in view of their risk, family goals, and ethical and religious standards and act in accordance with that decision
- Make the best possible psychological adjustment to the disorder in a family member and/or to the possible recurrence of the disorder

The most distinctive feature of genetic counseling is the nondirective approach, which does not seek to tell individuals what to do but to provide them with options and assist them with choosing the most appropriate course of action. The philosophy stems from the reaction against eugenics (see Chapter 1). A **directive approach**, which medical professionals are trained to provide, would be "Take this medication twice a day." A **nondirective approach** would be "There are two medications, each with its own side effects and benefits, to choose between. Or you can choose not to take any medication, and these conditions would be the consequences." Some patients prefer to be told what to do, and others wish to participate in the decision. Management issues tend to be handled in a more directive fashion when few options are available, but issues such as procreation choices, presymptomatic genetic testing, and acquisition of genetic information that affects multiple generations should be dealt with in a nondirective, noncoercive manner.

Genetic counseling may be performed by any trained health care professional but is more typically conducted by a genetic counselor with an advanced degree or by a physician who specializes in clinical genetics. Counselors and geneticists have completed a certified training or fellowship program and should have passed a board examination. Physician geneticists have also completed subspecialty training in one of any number of specialties, such as pediatrics, internal medicine, or obstetrics and gynecology, and are able to make appropriate diagnoses and prescribe therapy.

RISK ASSESSMENT BASED ON PEDIGREE ANALYSIS

Risk assessment is an important component of genetic counseling. It uses the individual's medical history, including the family medical history, and knowledge of mendelian inheritance patterns to determine the following:

- The approximate risk that a family will have another affected child
- The likelihood that an unaffected individual is capable of passing on a genetic abnormality to the next generation
- The likelihood that a person may develop a disease as an adult

Any medical practitioner should be able to make a basic risk assessment.

Chapter 7 discusses variations from the typical mendelian patterns that must also be considered to increase the validity of the risk assessment. Genetic counselors may also use a statistical method known as Bayesian analysis to determine how much the risk of recurrence is modified by disease prevalence, sensitivity and specificity of detection methods, and the numbers of affected or unaffected individuals in the family. As a result of genetic counseling, individuals may seek cytogenetic or genetic testing to contribute to the risk assessment or to assist in determining the appropriate management.

USMLE-style questions are not a good way to practice risk assessment. Open-ended discussion with colleagues is a better tool. For instance, Figure 6.9 shows a four-generation family pedigree. Not all affected individuals have a definitive diagnosis of a disease, and analysis of the symptoms within the family may help pinpoint the nature of the disorder.

- What is the likely inheritance pattern of the disorder shown in Fig 6.9?
  - If it is autosomal dominant, how can you explain III-3?
  - If it is autosomal recessive, how can you explain the presence of affected individuals in three different generations?
  - Is the gene for this disorder on the X or Y chromosome?
  - Is it possible to determine a single inheritance pattern from the information provided?
- Further questioning of the family reveals that the disease symptoms were present at birth in all affected individuals and that III-3 has no symptoms.
  - Does this help pinpoint the inheritance pattern any better?
- A literature search and use of on-line databases allow you to diagnose the family with a known autosomal recessive disorder.
  - Which individuals must be heterozygotes?
  - Which individuals are possible heterozygotes?

- What factors might contribute to the presence of so many heterozygotes for a disease with which you were not familiar?
- What is the frequency of heterozygotes in the general population for this disease?

HARDY-WEINBERG EQUILIBRIUM

In 1908, an English mathematician, Godfrey Hardy, and a German physician, Wilhelm Weinberg, independently presented observations on the effect of reproduction in a large population. The result, Hardy-Weinberg equilibrium, helps predict the distribution of phenotypes and genotypes in large populations. It is an approximation, because it represents an ideal situation in which a population is extremely large, all individuals reproduce, all mates are randomly selected, and all individuals have the same number of offspring. In addition, no circumstances that may disrupt the equilibrium are present; no new mutations occur, no selection for or against the genotype exists, and no migration is occurring in or out of the population. The traditional expression of the Hardy-Weinberg equilibrium involves two alleles, dominant and recessive, for any gene and does not consider multiple alleles or any nonmendelian influences.

Theory

To apply the Hardy-Weinberg principle, it helps to understand the basic derivation of the equilibrium. If two alleles are present, the sum of the frequency of the dominant alleles (p) and frequency of the recessive alleles (q) equals 1.

$$p + q = 1$$

Dominant alleles in genotypes are often referred to as A, homozygotes as AA, and heterozygotes as Aa. It is very difficult to measure the number of alleles in a population; therefore, it is approximated by the frequency of observed phenotypes. The number of dominant alleles in a population then may be approximated by

$$p = AA + 1/2\ Aa$$

where AA and Aa represent the total observed number of people with the dominant pheno-

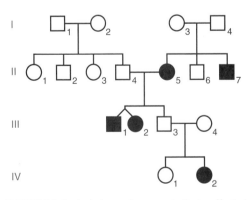

FIGURE 6.9 Dark circles and squares indicate affected individuals.

type. The specific distribution of AA and Aa cannot be determined by phenotypic observation alone. Conversely, the number of recessive alleles in a population is

$$q = 1/2 \text{ Aa} + \text{aa}$$

where aa represents the observed number of people with the recessive phenotype. Hardy and Weinberg determined that the phenotypic distribution could be predicted mathematically:

$$p + q = 1$$
$$(p + q)^2 = 1^2$$
$$p^2 + 2pq + q^2 = 1$$

or

$$\text{AA} + \text{Aa} + \text{aA} + \text{aa} = 100\%$$

Application

The Hardy-Weinberg equilibrium is helpful in clinical risk assessment because it provides a mechanism to convert an easily observable phenotypic frequency (aa) into a heterozygote carrier frequency for disorders inherited in a classic mendelian fashion. Heterozygote frequencies cannot otherwise be estimated by phenotypic observation but can be definitively determined only by expensive genotypic screening of large populations.

Again, refer to Figure 6.9. Individuals I-1, I-2, II-1, II-2, II-3, and II-4 all come from the same population, which has an observed aa frequency of 1 in 10,000.

- What is the likelihood that II-4 is a heterozygote (Aa)?

$$q^2 \text{ (or aa)} = 1/10{,}000$$
$$q = 1/100$$
$$p + q = 1; \text{ therefore } p = 1 - q$$
$$p = 99/100$$
$$2pq \text{ (or Aa)} = 2\,(99/100)\,(1/100)$$
$$2pq = 198/10{,}000 = 0.0198, \text{ or } 1.98\%$$

The carrier frequency in the population is approximately 2%.

If aa is very rare in the population, p can be assumed to be approximately 1, and the pre-ceding calculation can be further simplified:

$$2pq = 2\,(1)\,(1/100) = 1/50 = 0.02 \text{ or } 2\%$$

If aa is more common in the population, p should be used in the calculation. For example:

$$q^2 = 1/100$$
$$q = 1/10; \text{ therefore } p = 9/10$$
$$2pq = 2\,(9/10)\,(1/10) = 18/100 = 18\%$$

PRENATAL DIAGNOSIS OF MENDELIAN DISORDERS

Chorionic villus sampling, amniocentesis, and cordocentesis may all be used for the detection of chromosomal abnormalities as well as to obtain DNA for direct genetic testing of mendelian disorders. Direct genetic testing is used only if a mutation has been detected in the family. Some mendelian disorders may be detected prenatally through biochemical analysis of villus or amniocyte cultured cells. Prior to conception, families at risk for mendelian disorders should seek information from a maternal–fetal medicine specialist and genetic counselor to plan an appropriate testing strategy.

Some at-risk families do not wish to use routine prenatal diagnostic methods because of the gestational timing at diagnosis and the desire to avoid an affected pregnancy without resorting to termination of an affected fetus. For some of these families, preimplantation genetic diagnosis (PGD) is an option. However, PGD is expensive and relatively complex. PGD combines techniques of in vitro fertilization with molecular genetic techniques, such as fluorescence in situ hybridization and polymerase chain reaction, that are capable of diagnosing chromosomal or genetic abnormalities in as few as one or two cells.

In PGD, simultaneous development of multiple ova is stimulated with fertility drugs and monitored with ultrasonography. When appropriate, the ova are harvested with a transvaginal needle and ultrasonographic guidance. The ova are placed with sperm provided by the man or obtained by needle aspiration, and fertilization is allowed to take place (Fig. 6.10). The sperm may also be injected directly into the ova (intracytoplasmic

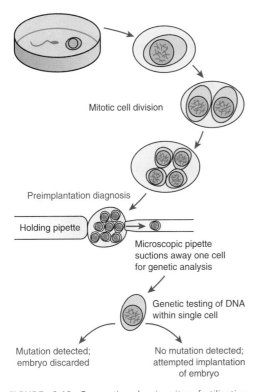

Mitotic cell division

Preimplantation diagnosis

Holding pipette

Microscopic pipette
suctions away one cell
for genetic analysis

Genetic testing of DNA
within single cell

Mutation detected;
embryo discarded

No mutation detected;
attempted implantation
of embryo

FIGURE 6.10 Conception by in vitro fertilization. Preimplantation genetic diagnosis can be performed only in the context of in vitro fertilization. Unaffected embryos are chosen for attempted implantation in the uterus but may be heterozygous carriers if the disorder is autosomal recessive. (Redrawn with permission from GeneTests: Medical Genetics Information Resource (database online). Educational Materials: Glossary. Copyright, University of Washington, Seattle, Washington, 1993–2005. Available at http://www.genetests.org.)

sperm injection). The fertilized embryos are monitored for the initiation of cell division. When the six- to eight-cell stage is reached, 2 to 3 days after fertilization, the zona pellucida surrounding the fertilized embryo is cut with a scalpel or laser and one to two cells are removed with a micropipette for molecular genetic analysis. Embryos that are determined to be unaffected by the disease in question are placed into the uterus under ultrasonographic guidance. A successful pregnancy occurs in 15 to 20% of attempts.

Some concern has been raised about the safety of all assisted reproduction technologies because of an increased incidence of imprinted disorders, specifically Beckwith-Wiedemann syndrome and Angelman syndrome, in children conceived by these methods. Is the imprinting mechanism disrupted by the technology? Both imprinting and the assisted reproduction are occurring during the same period in embryonic development.

ETHICS   Gender Selection in X-Linked Disorders

Although Western society places a value on a gender-balanced family, other cultures have a significant preference for sons. In some cultures, notably in northern India and China, the preference for sons may result in discrimination against daughters.

It is estimated that the Indian population has a deficit of approximately 50 million women for the three principal reasons historically given: (a) maternal death at childbirth, (b) enhanced nutritional and medical care for male offspring, and (c) female infanticide. Prenatal sex determination through ultrasonography and subsequent abortion of female fetuses has replaced infanticide and is thought by some to be occurring at an estimated annual rate of 2 million to 5 million in India alone, even with government prohibitions.

After China adopted the one-child policy as a method of population control for its burgeoning population, an increase in selective abortions, female infanticides, and abandonment of female infants has been observed, although official policy prohibits prenatal sex selection. Of the many Chinese infants left anonymously at orphanages and adopted by U.S. couples, virtually all are female. The gender ratio in China is now estimated to be 120 males to 100 females, compared to the naturally occurring ratio of 105:100.

Preimplantation sex selection has the potential to shift the gender selection mechanism from selective abortion and infanticide to assisted reproductive technologies. This mechanism may be more palatable for some cultures, which have religious or cultural objections to abortion yet advocate a specific gender balance in offspring. For instance, some schools of thought in Judaism state that the procreative responsibility of each family is to produce at least one son and one daughter, with a stronger emphasis on the son. Some define the time when life begins as later in gestation than the 2- to 4-day-old embryos studied in preimplantation diagnosis.

Various professional organizations have developed policies about gender selection. The World Health Organization has proposed ethical guidelines suggesting that only disease-related criteria should be used for prenatal gender selection, not fetal gender and paternity. The International Federation of Gynecology and Obstetrics (FIGO), the American College of Obstetricians and Gynecologists (ACOG), and the American Society of Reproductive Medicine (ASRM) have recommended ways their members should conduct themselves in regard to sex selection, particularly in preimplantation diagnosis and transfer of selected embryos.

In the West, the rights of the adult individual are given precedence, and many people feel that the rights of the parents to have an infant of a certain sex should be defended. Many couples wish to have a child of a specific gender to provide gender balance among existing children; they have no general preference for boys or girls. This practice is viewed as reproductive freedom.

When a family has been shown to carry an X-linked genetic abnormality, however, prenatal gender selection takes on a new significance, because of the likelihood that 50% of the sons of a carrier mother will be affected with the disease. Some families may choose to have more traditional methods of prenatal diagnosis, with the option to terminate an affected pregnancy if the disease is known to have a very severe phenotype. For those whose religious and cultural backgrounds distinguish between termination of an implanted pregnancy and selection of embryos prior to implantation, particularly some individuals from Jewish or Islamic traditions, PGD offers a previously unattainable option to have healthy children. (The Roman Catholic church does not favor either abortion or in vitro fertilization.)

Because there are far more X-linked recessive than X-linked dominant disorders, female carriers of X-linked disorders are most likely to have a normal phenotype. PGD can be performed even if a specific mutation was not detected in a gene. The embryos can be screened for gender, and only female embryos can be implanted. No male embryos would be implanted, so there would be no risk of implanting an affected male embryo. PGD for an X-linked disorder can be performed very accurately if a mutation of a known gene has been detected. In this situation, all four combinations can be distinguished—normal female, carrier female, normal male, and affected male. All embryos except the affected male embryos are suitable for implantation.

USMLE-Style Questions

1. Assume an autosomal recessive disorder with onset in infancy is demonstrated in the pedigree. Which of the following percentages is the likelihood that the adult represented by III-3 in the pedigree is a carrier of the recessive disorder?

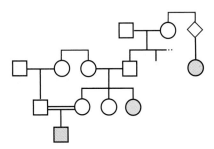

   a. 25%
   b. 33%
   c. 50%
   d. 67%
   e. 100%

2. Refer to Figure 6.9. If the disorder shown is an autosomal recessive disorder inherited in a standard mendelian fashion, which individuals must be heterozygotes?
   a. I-3, I-4, III-3, III-4
   b. I-3, I-4, II-4, III-3, III-4
   c. I-3, I-4, II-5, II-7, III-1, III-2, III-3, IV-2
   d. II-5, II-7, III-1, III-2, IV-2
   e. II-5, II-7, III-1, III-2, III-3, IV-2

3. A woman had a brother who died of Menkes disease, an X-linked recessive disorder of copper metabolism, at 2 years of age. Characteristics of the disease include unusual hair, seizures, mental retardation, and early death. She is planning to become pregnant and does not want to give birth to a son with Menkes disease. Prior to the child's death, no gene testing of the copper ATPase gene was performed. Prenatal testing is also available by biochemical analysis of fetal cells, but the copper defect is not expressed in amniocytes. Which of the following prenatal diagnostic methods should be used?
   a. Amniocentesis at 15 weeks
   b. Cordocentesis at 28 weeks
   c. Chorionic villus sampling at 11 weeks
   d. Preimplantation genetic diagnosis
   e. Ultrasonography at 18 weeks

SUGGESTED READINGS

Burke W. Genetic testing. N Engl J Med 2002;347:1867–1875.

Damewood MD. Ethical implications of a new application of preimplantation diagnosis. JAMA 2001;285:3143–3144.

Gosden R, Trasler J, Lucifero D, Faddy M. Rare congenital disorders, imprinted genes, and assisted reproductive technology. Lancet 2003;361:1975–1977.

Nagy AM, De Man X, Ruibal N, Lints FA. Scientific and ethical issues of preimplantation diagnosis. Ann Med 1998;30:1–6.

Towner D, Loewy RS. Ethics of preimplantation diagnosis for a woman destined to develop early-onset Alzheimer disease. JAMA 2002;287:1038–1040.

Vastag B. Merits of embryo screening debated. JAMA 2004;291:927–929.

WEB RESOURCES

http://www.ncbi.nlm.nih.gov/entrez/query.fcgi?db=OMIM

   Online Mendelian Inheritance in Man (OMIM) from Johns Hopkins University contains a search engine for disorders and genes that may be helpful. The clinical description of disorders is concise and the explanation of gene names informative. However, the accompanying literature review is presented in a chronological fashion rather than as a synthesis and can be contradictory and confusing.

http://www.ama-assn.org/ama/pub/category/2380.html

   The American Medical Association developed family history tools which may be downloaded. The Family Medical History in Disease Prevention pamphlet provides a physician or other health care provider with useful information about the utility of a family history in identifying disease risk and developing a personalized prevention program.

http://www.nsgc.org

   The web site of the National Society of Genetic Counselors has a consumer information section that contains a resource to locate genetic counselors across the United States and Canada.

http://www.asrm.org

   The Web site of the American Society of Reproductive Medicine has an Ethics Issues section that contains several position papers on gender selection and assisted reproductive technologies; they are reviewed regularly for continued appropriateness.

http://www.acog.org

   The Web site of the American College of Obstetrics and Gynecology has an Ethics in Ob-Gyn section that contains a variety of position papers.

http://www.figo.org

   The Web site of the International Federation of Gynecology and Obstetrics has an Ethical Guidelines section that contains a downloadable booklet, a 2003 collection of guidelines.

Unexpected Phenotypes in Mendelian Disorders: Molecular Explanations

Alice laughed. "There's no use in trying," she said. "One can't believe impossible things." "I daresay you haven't had much practice," said the Queen. "When I was your age, I always did it for half-an-hour a day. Why, sometimes I've believed as many as six impossible things before breakfast."

LEWIS CARROLL
Alice in Wonderland (1865)

Gregor Mendel's theories served as the infrastructure of observational medical genetics in the early to mid twentieth century. However, many diseases did not seem to be inherited according to the basic rules of autosomal versus X-linked and dominant versus recessive inheritance. The application of molecular genetics to these observations has begun to unlock these secrets and make sense of seemingly irrational findings.

VARIATIONS IN DOMINANT PHENOTYPES

Penetrance

It would make life easier for geneticists if a dominant disorder produced the same symptoms and severity of symptoms in every person who carried the dominant genotype. However, this is rarely the case. An individual may be a carrier of the genotype, as documented by either molecular analysis or family history, and not manifest the condition. The likelihood that a characteristic manifests itself is **penetrance,** and each dominant trait has a degree of penetrance that has been observed historically. The failure to manifest is **nonpenetrance,** which presents a dilemma regarding risk assessment. In the absence of molecular genotyping, does a person without symptoms have a normal genotype and no risk of transmitting an abnormal gene or have a nonpenetrant trait and a risk of transmitting the abnormal genotype? Nonpenetrance may cause the phenotype to skip a generation.

The reasons for nonpenetrance of a characteristic are many:

- Disorders may be expressed by individuals of only one sex. For example, a man may carry a mutation in his *BRCA1* gene that causes hereditary breast/ovarian cancer syndrome, but he cannot develop ovarian cancer and is not likely to develop breast cancer. If he transmits the mutated gene to his daughters, however, they may develop breast or ovarian

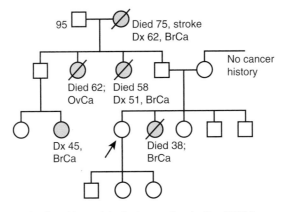

FIGURE 7.1 Pedigree from a family with an inherited mutation in the *BRCA1* gene, which causes hereditary breast/ovarian cancer syndrome. Penetrance does not occur in individuals II-1 and II-4 because of the sex-limited nature of the syndrome, but they are obligate carriers of the gene based on the appearance of the phenotype in their daughters. BrCa, breast cancer; OvCa, ovarian cancer.

cancer (Fig. 7.1). He is an **obligate carrier**—an individual who has a nonpenetrant condition and who *has* affected children.

- Disorders may not become evident until an individual has reached a certain age or been exposed to a specific environmental trigger. For example, a man with a genetic susceptibility to lung cancer may develop the disorder only if he is also exposed to the carcinogens in cigarette smoke, or a woman with a susceptibility to adult-onset diabetes mellitus may develop the disease only if her weight exceeds a certain threshold.

- Disorders that were once thought to be monogenic mendelian disorders are now known to be influenced by the presence of **modifier genes,** which may either increase or decrease (**protective alleles**) the penetrance of the disorder. This is discussed in greater detail in Chapter 9.

Variable Expressivity

Different features of a disorder may be evident in different members of the same family. This phenomenon, which is caused by the same factors that cause nonpenetrance, is known as **variable expressivity.**

Neurofibromatosis type I, a disorder noted for its variable expressivity within a family, is caused by a defect in the *NF1* gene on 17q11. *NF1* is very large (about 350 kilobases and 60 exons) and codes for at least three alternatively spliced transcripts. One of its introns contains

coding sequences for at least three other genes. The gene product, neurofibromin, interacts with the ras pathway, activates ras GTPase, and participates in the control of cellular proliferation; in addition, it likely has other functions yet to be determined. Clinical criteria have been developed to make the diagnosis and to emphasize the clinical variability of the disorder (Box 7.1). Some features may be present in early childhood (Fig. 7.2—see color insert),

---

BOX 7.1

Diagnostic Criteria for Neurofibromatosis Type I

Two or more of the following criteria must be present:

- Six or more café-au-lait spots of 0.5 cm (prepubertal) to more than 1.5 cm (postpubertal) diameter
- Two or more axillary or inguinal freckles
- Two or more Lisch nodules of iris
- Two or more neurofibromas or one plexiform neuroma
- Optic glioma
- Dysplasia of long bone, vertebrae, or base of skull
- First-degree relative with neurofibromatosis

and others may appear over time. Some individuals have as few as two small lesions of the nerve endings (neurofibromas) and others have hundreds. Penetrance of neurofibromatosis is nearly complete; individuals with an *NF1* mutation almost always exhibit some features of the disease. There is a lack of genotype–phenotype correlation among families, and the variable expressivity observed within a family points to the action of modifier genes as well as sporadic alterations of somatic cells that modify the disease phenotype.

Anticipation (see Chapter 5) is a specific type of variable expressivity caused by the instability of triplet microsatellite repeat regions. With successive generations, the severity of a disease may worsen, and the age of onset may decrease. The myotonic dystrophies may be diagnosed from adulthood to infancy. Symptoms may be as mild as cataracts and myotonia (decreased ability to release a muscle contraction and initiate a new contraction) and as serious as severe hypotonia and respiratory insufficiency in the newborn. Type 1 (DM1) is caused by an increase in the CTG repeat in the 3′ untranslated region of the *DMPK* gene (*d*ystrophia *m*yotonica–*p*rotein

*k*inase) on 19q13 (see Fig. 5.7). The CTG repeat size is well correlated to clinical phenotype and age of onset (Table 7.1), although some overlap occurs. Type 2 (DM2) is caused by an untranslated CCTG expansion in intron 1 of the zinc finger protein-9 gene (*ZNF9*) at 3q13.3-q24, with alleles ranging in size from 75 to 11,000 CCTG repeats; the mean is 5000 repeats. The repeats that cause both DM1 and DM2 are translated into RNA but do not alter the coding region of the gene. A gain of function at the RNA level with accumulation of the repeat-containing transcripts in the nucleus and interference with the RNA-binding proteins involved in RNA splicing is hypothesized.

De Novo Mutations

Dominant mutations are present in multiple successive generations in some disorders and in some families. The original mutation had to occur spontaneously at some time in the past. When a **de novo mutation,** or new mutation, of a dominant characteristic first occurs, it is not possible to use the existing family history to determine the inheritance pattern. From that

TABLE 7.1 CORRELATION OF PHENOTYPE AND CTG REPEAT SIZE IN MYOTONIC DYSTROPHY

PHENOTYPE	CLINICAL SIGNS	CTG REPEAT SIZE (SOME OVERLAP BETWEEN PHENOTYPES)	AGE OF ONSET (YEARS)
Normal	None	38–~49	(not applicable)
Mild	Cataracts	50–~150	20–70
	Mild myotonia		
Classic	Weakness	~100 to ~1000–1500	10–30
	Myotonia		
	Cataracts		
	Balding		
	Cardiac arrhythmia		
	Others		
Congenital	Infantile hypotonia	~1000 to >2000	Birth to 10
	Respiratory deficits		
	Mental retardation		

Adapted from T. Bird (Updated 2004). Myotonic Dystrophy Type I. In GeneReviews at GeneTests: Medical Genetics Information Resource (database online). Copyright, University of Washington, Seattle, Washington, 1997–2005. Available at http://www.genetests.org.

point on, however, the characteristic exhibits a standard mendelian inheritance pattern.

Some genes or specific locations within genes have a particularly high rate of new mutations. The larger the coding region of a gene, the more likely it is to mutate by chance. The *NF1* gene is a frequent location for de novo mutations, which is not surprising, given the extremely large size of the gene. Genes with regions of methylated CG dinucleotides are likely to have de novo mutations because of cytosine deamination.

On occasion, a specific nucleotide exhibits a predisposition for mutation. The purine guanine at position 1138 of the fibroblast growth factor receptor 3 gene (*FGFR3*) on 4p16.3 spontaneously changes to the purine adenine or to the pyrimidine cytosine in 2.8 of every 10,000 births. The G → A nucleotide transition occurs in 98% of cases. Either change results in a G380R (glycine → arginine) missense mutation in the FGFR3 protein and causes achondroplasia, the most common type of dwarfism (Fig. 7.3). FGFR3, which is normally expressed in chondrocytes at the growth plate of developing long bones, inhibits excessive growth. The G380R mutation is a gain-of-function mutation that causes constitutive activation of the FGFR3 protein, further increasing the growth inhibition, probably through increased apoptosis of chondrocytes. As with other de novo dominant mutations, an individual with this mutation who has unaffected parents still has a 50% chance of having an affected child. It is fairly common for two individuals with achondroplasia to have children. Prenatal diagnosis is used to diagnose homozygous achondroplasia, which occurs in 25% of offspring of these couples. Infants who are homozygous for the G380R mutation have severe disruption of bone growth and do not typically survive the neonatal period.

Some dominant disorders are lethal in the neonatal or early childhood period and therefore never occur as the result of inheritance from an affected parent. De novo mutation is the sole source of these disorders, and the likelihood of recurrence in any family is the same as the risk of having a new mutation occur again. One example is thanatophoric

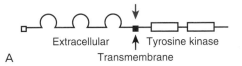

A

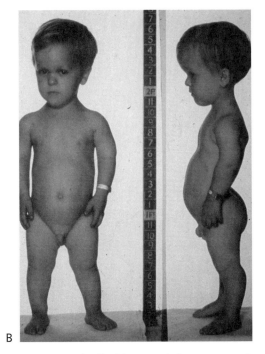

B

FIGURE 7.3 A. The fibroblast growth factor receptor 3 protein has three immunoglobulin-like extracellular domains responsible for ligand binding, a transmembrane domain, and two intracellular tyrosine kinase domains. The missense mutation responsible for more than 99% of achondroplasia occurs at position 380 in the transmembrane portion (blue arrow). **B.** A child with achondroplasia due to a G380R mutation in the transmembrane portion of *FGFR3*. He shows the large head circumference, frontal bossing, disproportionate shortening of the proximal long bones (rhizomelic pattern), and lumbar lordosis. Intelligence is normal. Average adult height is 125 to 130 cm (49 to 51 inches). (Part B from *Pediatrics* (1984) by Booth and Wezniak. Distributed in the United States by Williams & Wilkins for Gower Medical. Image 45.)

(death bearing) dysplasia, a micromelic form of dwarfism resulting in death in the first hours of life. Ribs and long bones are extremely short, and the skin of the extremities appears in redundant folds. Vertebral bodies are greatly reduced in height and are **H**-shaped on anteroposterior radiographs. Type 1 thanatophoric dysplasia is associated with short bowed femurs shaped like 1960s-era telephone receivers and sometimes with a normal head shape or a skull shaped like a three-leafed clover (cloverleaf skull). Type 2 thanatophoric dysplasia is associated with somewhat longer but straighter femurs and always with a severe cloverleaf skull (Fig. 7.4). Cloverleaf skull is due to premature fusion of cranial sutures (craniosynostosis). Both types 1 and 2 thanatophoric dysplasia are associated with gain-of-function mutations in the *FGFR3* gene, with even more apoptosis of chondrocytes than is observed in achondroplasia.

Mosaicism

When de novo mutations are observed in children of unaffected parents, it is possible that the mutation originated spontaneously in the parental gamete. It may also have originated as a somatic mutation during embryogenesis in the parent (see Chapter 3). The population of mutated cells may be too small to cause an observable phenotype in the parent. If the mutation involves somatic cells only, there is no risk to future generations (**somatic mosaicism**). If the mutation involves germline cells (**germline or gonadal mosaicism**), the risk to the next generation may be as high as if the parent had the disorder. The initial family history may resemble that with an autosomal recessive disorder, with multiple affected siblings and unaffected parents (Fig. 7.5). The rate of germline mosaicism may be as high as 5 to 15% in a seem-

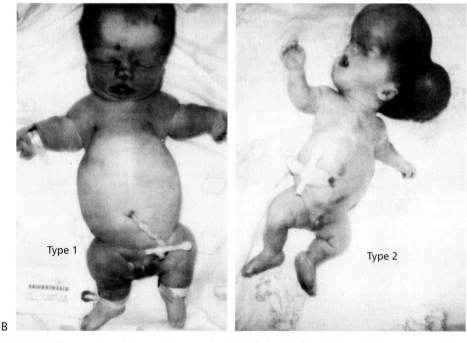

FIGURE 7.4 A. Stillborn infant with type 1 thanatophoric dysplasia. **B.** Infant delivered stillborn at term with type 2 thanatophoric dysplasia. Both type 1 and type 2 are associated with gain-of-function mutations in the *FGFR3* gene. Type 1 is caused by various missense mutations in the extracellular domain, all of which result in the addition of a cysteine which probably causes constitutive dimerization of two FGFR3 proteins (blue bracket). Type 2 is caused by a single missense mutation (lys650glu or K650E) in the tyrosine kinase domain (blue arrow). Compare the relative limb shortening in these infants with the child in Figure 7.3.

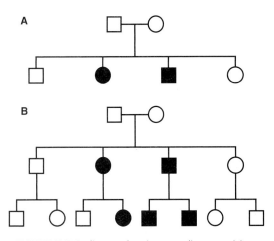

FIGURE 7.5 Pedigrees showing germline mosaicism. Germline mosaicism may be difficult to discern (**A**) until the next generation has been observed (**B**). Many dominant disorders have appeared in older literature as also having a "recessive" form. These recessive forms have frequently been reclassified as germline mosaicism when additional generations were born.

ingly new disorder. This possibility must be incorporated into the recurrence risk assessment provided to families.

Genetic mosaicism is inevitable. Postzygotic mutations are an expected and unavoidable occurrence. Germline mosaicism occurs when the postzygotic mutation takes place in early embryogenesis, as the gamete progenitors are established. Somatic mosaicism may occur at any time in the life of the individual and is an important contributor to disease development (see Chapter 8).

Genetic Heterogeneity

Genetic heterogeneity may also complicate phenotypic and genotypic analysis. **Clinical heterogeneity** occurs when mutations in the same gene produce different clinical disorders. Examples that have already been discussed include the *RET* gene (MEN2 and Hirschsprung disease) and the *FGFR3* gene (achondroplasia and thanatophoric dysplasia types 1 and 2). **Allelic heterogeneity** occurs when multiple mutations within the same allele cause a disorder. Most disorders caused by loss-of-function mutations exhibit allelic heterogeneity. Many phenotypes are caused by **locus heterogeneity**; that is, mutations at

more than one gene locus. Examples include *FANC* complementation groups (Fanconi anemia) and *BRCA1* and *BRCA2* (hereditary breast/ovarian cancer syndrome).

Phenocopy

Another complication is the occurrence within a family of a phenotype that is similar to a particular disorder but developed in the absence of an inherited genotype. These **phenocopies** are seen frequently in adult-onset disorders such as cancer. For example, a woman may develop breast cancer in a family with hereditary breast/ovarian cancer syndrome through a mechanism completely unrelated to any inherited defect in the *BRCA1* or *BRCA2* genes.

Parent-of-Origin Effect

Most disorders or characteristics that have a parent-of-origin effect are inherited in a dominant fashion (see Chapter 4). Interpretation of family histories of imprinted characteristics or disorders may be very difficult (Figs. 7.6 to 7.8) and requires multigenerational histories with large sibships for adequate analysis.

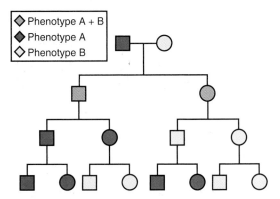

FIGURE 7.6 Pedigree showing inheritance of two separate characteristics in an extended family. Each characteristic is encoded by a gene for which parent-of-origin (or imprinting) is a factor. The genes are at separate loci, but one is paternally imprinted (maternally expressed) and one is maternally imprinted (paternally expressed). For clarity the characteristics have been shown at a highly improbable 100% transmission rate from generation II onward. (All individuals in generations II, III, and IV inherit genes for both characteristics.) Phenotype A is maternally imprinted (paternal expression). Phenotype B is paternally imprinted (maternal expression).

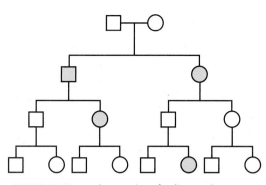

FIGURE 7.7 Paternal expression of a disease phenotype. The mutated gene must be inherited from the father to be expressed. The mother may pass on the mutated gene, but it will be imprinted in her children and have no phenotypic effect until future generations. The likelihood of the mutated gene being transmitted to a child is 50% for any conception.

Knowledge of the molecular basis of parent-of-origin effects allows practitioners to provide a more complete risk assessment to families. For instance, an infant diagnosed with Beckwith-Wiedemann syndrome may have molecular diagnostic testing to determine whether the disorder is caused by uniparental disomy disrupting the imprinting pattern, chromosomal microdeletion of the region, or point mutation disrupting imprinting. An infant diagnosed with uniparental disomy as the cause should have no risk of transmitting the disorder, because the uniparental

disomy is highly unlikely to recur. Similarly, the infant's parents have a negligible risk of having another affected child. An infant diagnosed with either a microdeletion or a point mutation has a 50% risk of transmitting the abnormal gene, but expression in the next generation is determined by the infant's gender (maternal expression). The infant's parents can be tested for the abnormality to determine whether they have a 50% risk of having another affected child. It may not be possible, however, to determine whether either parent has germline mosaicism.

VARIATIONS IN RECESSIVE PHENOTYPES

Frequently Occurring Alleles

If a recessive allele occurs commonly in a population, there is an increased likelihood that recessive traits may appear in multiple generations of a family. Sickle cell disease is one of the most common autosomal recessive disorders and is the most common inherited blood disorder in the United States. It is caused by an E6V (glutamine → valine) mutation in the β-globin protein, which forms a unique hemoglobin (Hb S). In deoxygenated Hb S, the added valine interacts with regions on adjacent molecules and undergoes intracytoplasmic polymerization and aggregation that distort the red blood cells, resulting in sickling, as well as damaging the red cell membrane. The sickle cells are brittle, poorly able to alter their shape to negotiate small-caliber vascular beds, and prone to rupture or hemolysis. The homozygous condition is sickle cell disease, and the relatively asymptomatic heterozygous condition is sickle cell trait. The E6V allele is common in individuals who originate from Africa, India, the Mediterranean region, the Middle East, the Caribbean region, and parts of Central and South America. These areas have a high incidence of malaria, and sickle trait is thought to provide some protection against the infection. The prevalence of sickle cell disease in the United States is directly related to the ethnic background (Fig. 7.9). Sickle cell trait is present in 8 to 14% of African Americans and in as many as 25 to 30% of individuals who have re-

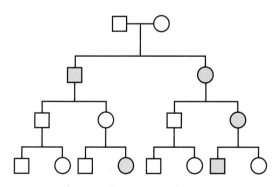

FIGURE 7.8 Maternal expression of a disease phenotype. The mutated gene must be inherited from the mother to be expressed. The father may pass on the mutated gene, but it will be imprinted in his children and have no phenotypic effect until future generations. The likelihood of the mutated gene being transmitted to a child is 50% for any conception.

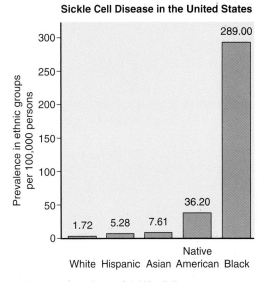

FIGURE 7.9 Prevalence of sickle cell disease among various U.S. ethnic groups. The prevalence range among African Americans has been given as 250 to 600 per 100,000. (Modified from www.fda.gov/fdac/features/496_sick.html.)

cently immigrated from West Africa. With such a high carrier frequency, there is a good probability that more than one carrier may partner with members of a heterozygous family, permitting homozygous individuals to be present in a pattern that may more closely mimic a dominant pedigree.

Founder Populations

The characteristics of the population may influence the frequency of an allele, particularly if the choice of mate is restricted by racial, ethnic, religious, or geographic boundaries. Some populations have an increased prevalence of some genetic mutations because of a **founder effect,** in which a small number of founding individuals, only one of whom may have had a genetic mutation, originates a population that is limited in some way. For instance, a few Jews (Ashkenazi) migrated to Eastern Europe after the separation of the Jewish peoples in Palestine in 70 A.D. For hundreds of years, they lived in small communities, and intermarriage with non-Jews was minimal. In addition, several times the population was bottlenecked, that is, significantly reduced through disease or violence, and

a few individuals emerged after the experience to reestablish local populations. The initial founder effect, subsequent cultural isolation, and bottlenecks led to an increased number of recessive disorders in the population (Box 7.2). Ashkenazi Jews also have an increased likelihood to have the dominant disorders hereditary breast/ovarian cancer syndrome and Machado Joseph disease, a triplet repeat disorder. The Jewish population which initially migrated around the shores of the Mediterranean Sea is Sephardic and is at risk for β-thalassemia, familial Mediterranean fever, glucose-6-phosphate dehydrogenase deficiency, and glycogen storage disorder type III.

Most of the Jewish population in the United States has Ashkenazi heritage. The increased risk of recessive disorders is well known, and several centers have been established to assist with carrier testing. Some groups of Orthodox Jews use the results of carrier testing to prevent arranged marriages between two individuals who are heterozygous for the same disorders.

BOX 7.2

Recessive Disorders More Common in Ashkenazi Jews

- Bloom syndrome
- Canavan disease
- Cystic fibrosis
- Fabry disease (α-galactosidase A deficiency; X-linked)
- Factor XI deficiency
- Familial dysautonomia
- Familial Mediterranean fever
- Fanconi anemia
- Gaucher disease (acid β-glucosidase deficiency)
- Mucolipidosis IV
- Neurosensory deafness (*DFNB1*)
- Niemann-Pick disease
- Nonclassic 21-hydroxylase deficiency
- Tay-Sachs disease (hexosaminidase A deficiency)
- Torsion dystonia

BOX 7.3

Recessive Disorders Common in the Amish from Holmes County, Ohio

- Ataxia-telangiectasia
- Cartilage-hair hypoplasia
- Cystic fibrosis
- Familial craniosynostosis
- Hemophilia B (factor IX deficiency; X-linked)
- Mast syndrome (late-onset spastic paraplegia)
- Microcephalic osteodysplastic primordial dwarfism type I
- Phenylketonuria
- Thyroid dysgenesis
- Troyer syndrome (early-onset progressive spastic paraplegia)

The smaller the number of founders, the more profound the effect may be on the community. Consider the Amish, who fled religious persecution in Switzerland and other parts of Europe in the 1700s and began migrating to North America. Different migratory waves settled in various parts of Pennsylvania and Ohio and did not necessarily mingle with established Amish communities. Twenty-one founder families eventually settled in Holmes County, Ohio, in the early 1800s in what has become the largest community of Amish in the world (approximately 24,000 in 2000). Religious and cultural isolation has led to genetic isolation in the Amish, who do not typically recruit new members through marriage or proselytizing and have limited geographic mobility because of their continued reliance on transportation without motors. Like Ashkenazi Jews, the Amish have an increased likelihood of having recessive disorders (Box 7.3), but the disorders are not the same. In fact, the disorders of the Holmes County Amish are different from those in Amish people who live in Lancaster County, Pennsylvania, the second largest Amish community.

Gene Expression Level

The phenotype of recessive disorders may also be influenced by the level of expression of the gene and the amount of functional protein produced. Classic 21-hydroxylase deficiency (21-OHD), or congenital adrenal hyperplasia, involves impaired synthesis of cortisol from its cholesterol precursor in the adrenal cortex (Fig. 7.10). Side effects are

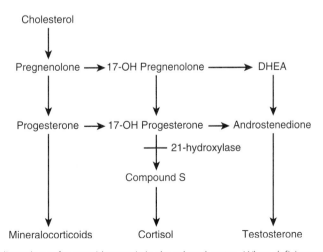

FIGURE 7.10 Metabolic pathway for steroidogenesis in the adrenal cortex. When deficiency of an enzyme is present in a biochemical path, a damlike effect causes precursor molecules to build up on one side and spill over into alternative pathways (such as androgen production) or be present in inadequate amounts in other pathways (aldosterone production).

excessive androgen synthesis, which produces virilization in all patients but is particularly noticeable in newborn girls as a cause of ambiguous genitalia (Fig. 7.11), and inadequate production of aldosterone, which may result in salt wasting, potentially life threatening in the first 4 weeks of life. Treatment is replacement of the deficient cortisol. Many states include screening for 21-OHD as part of the newborn screening panel, because 21-OHD in males is not readily apparent on physical examination. Classic 21-OHD is caused primarily by nonsense, frameshift, or splice site mutations of the *CYP21A2* gene on 6p21.3 or by large deletions of all or part of the gene that result in less than 10% enzyme activity. Salt wasting is associated with no enzyme activity at all and is present in 75% of those with classic 21-OHD.

Some individuals with 21-OHD have two missense mutations of *CYP21A2* or are compound heterozygotes with a severe mutation on one allele and a mild mutation on the other. The activity of the enzyme in these individuals is 20 to 50% of normal. The non-classic phenotype is milder, with no prenatal virilization or salt wasting, but symptoms of excessive androgen levels may appear at any time after birth. In adult females with non-classic 21-OHD, about 60% have hirsutism (increased hair growth) alone, about 10% hirsutism and abnormal menses, and about 10% abnormal menses alone. Fertility is low (approximately 50%), and many women develop polycystic ovaries. Males with non-classic 21-OHD may have early beard growth and an enlarged penis with relatively small testes. Treatment is not always necessary but may be done with cortisol at a lower dose than is needed for classic 21-OHD. The most common autosomal recessive disorder in Ashkenazi Jews is nonclassic 21-OHD, which occurs in 1 in 27 (3.7%) of the Jewish population. It is also increased in Hispanics, Slavs, and Italians and estimated to be present in 1% of the residents of New York City.

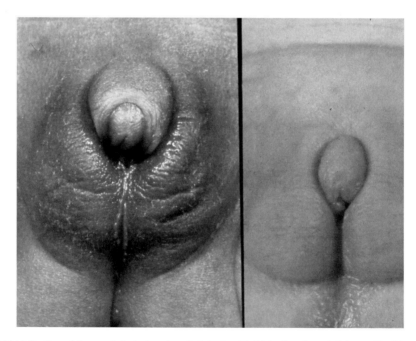

FIGURE 7.11 Virilization of the genitalia in two female infants with 21-hydroxylase deficiency. Physicians in delivery rooms may inadvertently assign an inappropriate gender to these infants. Testes are not palpable in the labioscrotal folds, which should provide the clue to the actual gender of the infant. (Reprinted with permission from *Slide Atlas of Pediatric Physical Diagnosis*: Gower Medical Publishing Ltd, 1987. Image 9.19C and D from Pediatric Endocrinology. Courtesy of Dr. D Becker.)

Consanguinity

Consanguineous individuals are more likely than the general population to share the same unique genotype and therefore are more likely to have children who may be homozygous and express an autosomal recessive phenotype. Some cultures promote marriages between cousins, particularly cultures that advocate arranged marriages. Some founder populations, such as the Amish, which do not actively seek partners outside their group (**inbred**), have high degrees of relatedness.

VARIATIONS IN X-LINKED PHENOTYPES

De novo mutations and germline mosaicism do not occur exclusively in dominant disorders. They are commonly found in X-linked disorders as well, both dominant and recessive.

Frequently Occurring Alleles

X-linked recessive disorders may also appear in unusual patterns in the pedigree if the allele occurs commonly. Glucose-6-phosphate dehydrogenase (G6PD) deficiency is the most common enzyme deficiency in the world; it affects an estimated 400 million individuals. G6PD is the first step of the hexose monophosphate shunt pathway that provides the sole source of NADPH for mature red blood cells, which lack the citric acid cycle. NADPH is essential to keep glutathione in its reduced form to protect the cell from oxidative stress. Red blood cells are at increased risk for oxidative stress because of their function and their lack of the citric acid cycle. In G6PD deficiency, stressed cells have an increased rate of hemolysis, which may cause anemia and jaundice. Hemolytic crises may be triggered by acute oxidative stresses produced by agents with strong oxidative properties, drugs (Box 7.4), infection, or the ingestion of fava beans.

G6PD deficiency is most prevalent in individuals from Africa, the Middle East, and Southeast Asia. The *G6PD* gene is at Xq28. Approximately 400 variants and mutations are known, almost all of which are point mutations or in-frame deletions of a small number of

---

BOX 7.4

Drugs Associated With Hemolysis in G6PD deficiency

- Aspirin
- Antimalarials
- Ascorbic acid
- Chloramphenicol
- Hydralazine
- Mestranol
- Methyldopa
- Nalidixic acid
- Nitrofurantoin
- Procainamide
- Quinidine
- Sulfonamides and sulfones
- Vitamin K (water soluble)

---

codons. The most ancient variant is asn126asp, which originated in Africa. A second mutation in this variant occurred within the last 10,000 years (val68met, asn126asp); known as G6PD A–, it resulted in a deleterious effect, with an 8 to 20% G6PD activity level and presence of disease phenotype. Both mutations must be present for the G6PD-deficient phenotype to manifest. The A– variant accounts for 20 to 40% of the affected population of western and central Africa and confers some malaria resistance to both affected males and carrier females. Approximately 10 to 14% of the male African American population exhibits G6PD deficiency.

Another common mutation, ser188phe, known as the Mediterranean variant, arose independently in both Europe and Asia, and it accounts for most disease in Italy, Greece, the Middle East, India, and Pakistan. The activity level of the enzyme is below 5%. This variant has an ability to interact with a second milder disorder, Gilbert (pronounced zhee-BEAR) syndrome, to produce a severe phenotype. Some infants with G6PD deficiency of the Mediterranean type develop severe neonatal hyperbilirubinemia, which allows deposition of unconjugated bilirubin pigment in the basal ganglia of the brain (kernicterus), resulting in cerebral palsy and mental retardation. Gilbert syndrome is a mild fluctuating elevation of bilirubin with normal liver enzymes caused by a variant in the *UGT1A1* gene on 2q37, which encodes for a member of the UDP-glycosyltransferase 1 family. The *UGT1* gene contains at least 12 ligand-specific promoters/exon 1 units, which are differentially spliced onto exons 2 through 5, forming the catalytic site for UDP-glucuronic acid. The A1 promoter/exon 1 subunit is thought to bind specifically to bilirubin. The two must be brought into proximity to allow appropriate conjugation of bilirubin, hence excretion.

Individuals of European origin with Gilbert syndrome are homozygous for an extra TA dinucleotide inserted in the TATAA promoter upstream of the gene, which results in reduced gene expression. Infants with the Mediterranean form of G6PD deficiency who are either heterozygous or homozygous for the promoter variant associated with Gilbert syndrome have a much higher rate of neonatal hyperbilirubinemia (30–50% versus 9%), and kernicterus or even death may result. Neither the G6PD deficiency nor the *UGT1A1* variant alone results in an increased rate of neonatal hyperbilirubinemia. This is an example of a relatively benign variant serving as a significant modifier gene.

Women who carry the G6PD mutation may or may not show any increase in hemolysis or mild hyperbilirubinemia, which depends in part on X-inactivation patterns (see Chapter 4). The natural somatic mosaicism of all women has a great influence on the expression of X-linked phenotypes. Examples of the effect of X-inactivation patterns are the creatine kinase levels in female carriers of Duchenne muscular dystrophy and factor VIII levels in female carriers of hemophilia A described in Chapter 4.

Male Lethality

X-linked disorders with a more dominant phenotype may appear to affect many more females than males, particularly if the phenotype in males is so severe that it is lethal.

Incontinentia pigmenti (IP) has a lethal male phenotype and is caused by a defect in the *IKBKG* gene at Xq28. The gene partially overlaps the *G6PD* gene at Xq28 and is transcribed in the opposite direction. It encodes for IKKγ and blocks the apoptotic effects of tumor necrosis factor. Affected females have a vesicular rash in the first few months of life that follows the lines of Blaschko; the vesicles disappear, but the area becomes hyperpigmented, fading during adolescence (Fig. 7.12—see color insert). Most individuals (80%) with IP have a deletion of exons 4 to 10 of the gene which occurred de novo during a paternal meiosis. The severely shortened IKKγ protein does not complex with two other proteins, which allows excessive apoptosis of cells, a lethal condition. Females with IP have skewed X-inactivation, in which the X chromosome with the mutant allele is preferentially inactivated. Living males with IP have been reported; they are somatic mosaics or have a 47,XXY karyotype. However, a few males have less severe mutations, such as a duplication of a 7-cytosine tract of exon 10 or a mutation of a stop codon permitting several additional amino acids; females with the same mutations have a milder phenotype.

Women with IP have a higher than usual risk of pregnancy loss due to the low viability of male fetuses. At delivery, the expected sex ratio of offspring is 33% unaffected females, 33% affected females, and 33% unaffected males. All X-linked disorders with male lethality have a similar sex ratio.

MITOCHONDRIAL INHERITANCE

Some families with affected individuals in multiple generations were assumed to have an X-linked dominant disorder because it was transmitted exclusively by mothers. However, affected males never passed the disorder on to their daughters, as would be expected. A mitochondrially inherited condition can affect both sexes but may be transmitted only by affected mothers. The 37 mitochondrial genes encoded by mitochondrial DNA (mtDNA) account for only a portion of the gene products used within the mitochondria, and most are encoded in the nucleus. Thus, disorders of mitochondrial energy production show a mixed inheritance pattern of recessive (nuclear origin) and matrilineal (mitochondrial origin).

The mitochondria in the newly fertilized ovum are thought to be almost exclusively maternal. The mitochondria of the sperm are densely packed at the neck of the sperm and provide the energy for the movement of the tail. Those that enter the cytoplasm of the egg at fertilization are preferentially destroyed by the proteosomes; hence the matrilineal inheritance of mtDNA.

Mitochondrial inheritance may also be complicated by a mixed population of normal and abnormal mitochondrial genomes within each cell (**heteroplasmy**), a specialized form of mosaicism. The egg may be heteroplasmic initially, and the passive random segregation of mitochondria during cell division may create cell and tissue types that have highly variable proportions of normal and abnormal genomes. In addition, the enhanced mutability of the mitochondrial genome may contribute to even more heteroplasmy during the life of the individual.

Disorders caused by mitochondrial genome mutations may be expressed according to the dosage of abnormal genomes present in the cell or tissue as well as interaction with polymorphisms and modifier genes. These combine to permit a wide range of perceived nonpenetrance and variable expression in affected families. In addition, the same genotype may produce very different phenotypes, depending on the accompanying factors and tissue prevalence.

Leber hereditary optic neuropathy is a mitochondrially inherited disorder with both gender- and age-dependent penetrance. Men tend to develop blurring and loss of central vision in their 20s. Women may be more severely affected, although they tend to develop symptoms later in life. In fact, the mother of a newly diagnosed man may not yet have developed symptoms herself. Most affected individuals (90–95%) have one of three point mutations in any of three respiratory chain components in the mtDNA, and 15% have heteroplasmy. Affected individuals usually have more than 75% abnormal mitochondria in white blood cells. Affected males do not transmit the mutation to any of their offspring, but affected females transmit it to all of their offspring. Penetrance is highly variable, with failure to develop symptoms in over 50% of men and 85% of women with mutations. Penetrance also depends somewhat on the specific mutation.

In most mitochondrial disorders, the genotype–phenotype correlation is poorly understood. It is better to remember the nature of the energy production of the mitochondria and its effect on highly aerobic tissues such as the nervous system and cardiac and skeletal muscle. Two disorders with mitochondrial inheritance that epitomize the multisystem nature of mitochondrial dysfunction are myoclonic epilepsy and ragged red fibers (MERRF) and myopathy, encephalopathy, lactic acidosis, and stroke-like episodes (MELAS). More than 90% of individuals with MERRF have a point mutation in the $tRNA^{lys}$ gene in mtDNA, and more than 95% of those with MELAS have a point mutation in the mtDNA $tRNA^{leu}$ gene. Proteins with large numbers of lysine or leucine residues are not synthesized well, and blockage in the respiratory chain process produces elevation in lactate and pyruvate in both disorders. Ragged red fibers are found on muscle biopsy in both MERRF and MELAS (Fig. 7.13).

FALSE PATERNITY

Unexpected or false paternity discovered in the course of genetic testing is a significant complication to phenotype and pedigree analysis. The true incidence of false paternity is unknown but ranges from 1 to 30% in various reports, with substantial differences in various socioeconomic and geographic locations. A disruption in the paternal lineage may occur for a number of reasons:

- Pregnancy outside of marriage
- Pregnant woman married a man who was not the father of her child

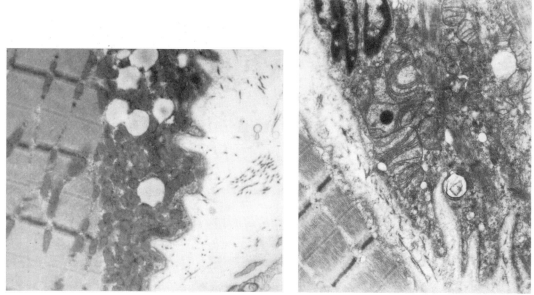

A   B

FIGURE 7.13 Electron micrographs of muscle biopsy in individual with mitochondrial myopathy. The striated skeletal muscle fibers with large collections of abnormally shaped mitochondria gathered at the periphery are seen on the left of each image. These large collections of abnormal mitochondria give the appearance of ragged red fibers on standard light microscopy. (Courtesy of Dr. T Prior, the Ohio State University Department of Pathology, Columbus, Ohio.)

- Adoption (formal or informal)
- Children known by stepfather's surname
- Uses of aliases
- Single mother with no attributed father
- Artificial insemination with donated sperm
- Identity error shortly after birth by health care institution

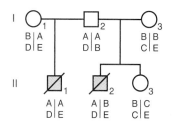

FIGURE 7.14 Genetic linkage analysis, or tracking of polymorphisms in the vicinity of the causative gene, may be used in families for whom direct mutation analysis is not possible. Linkage analysis of this family indicates that individual I-2 cannot be the father of individual II-3. In this setting, additional polymorphisms at other genetic loci would be studied to confirm false paternity.

On some occasions, the nonpaternity is well known to the family but was simply not reported to the health care practitioner. On other occasions, one or two family members may be aware of the nonpaternity but have not made it widely known. Rarely, the false paternity is a complete surprise to all family members.

Blood type analysis was used historically for analysis but is no longer considered adequate. In fact, some rare blood types lead less well trained individuals to conclude false paternity when that is not the case. (A case study is provided on the Web site.) Genetic testing using polymorphisms, similar to that used for forensic analyses, is an excellent means of resolving paternity issues, as it is unambiguous in its results. Many commercial laboratories offer paternity testing; unfortunately, the laboratories operate outside of the clinical certification process, and no national certification exists to ensure quality and accuracy of results.

ETHICS A Case of Unexpected Paternity: Should Genetic Counselors Reveal All Information?

Genetic testing may be performed on entire family groups during testing for presymptomatic adult-onset disorders or searching for a related living organ donor, as in the case of kidney transplantation. Nonpaternity may be discovered inadvertently and may have no bearing on the medical situation or the question being asked by the family. In that case the practitioner must balance the bioethical principles of patient autonomy (right to know) with nonmaleficence (do no harm).

Consider the following case: Matt and Sheila have a child, Ryan, with a severe autosomal recessive disorder. The family participates in a research study in which direct sequencing of Ryan's gene does not reveal an identifiable point mutation, but the family is found to have unique polymorphisms in the region that track with the disease. Unfortunately, Ryan dies of complications of his disease, and the stress on the family pushes Matt and Sheila into a divorce. Then Matt meets and marries Jodie. Their first child has the same autosomal recessive disorder, and the polymorphisms track with the disease. A second child is conceived, but the couple does not want prenatal diagnosis. At birth, their new daughter Abby appears healthy. Blood is obtained to check for the polymorphisms. The result, when it returns in 4 weeks, is surprising (Fig. 7.14).

When you meet with the couple to give them Abby's result, Matt starts the discussion by saying that he has never been happier. "Abby is such a joy! I've never had a child before who was so active. She's the light of my life. Tell me, Doc, is she going to develop symptoms, too?"

There is no easy answer to this dilemma. Most practitioners would not blurt out a statement of false paternity in this setting but would answer the question that Matt asked. "No, she doesn't have the disease. She's not even a carrier." Some would speak to Jodie privately and inform her that Abby has a different father, and others would not pursue the topic. If the interpretation of the test information is recorded in the medical record, it should ultimately be discussed with the family. If the family requested the medical records in the future and the practitioner had not made a complete disclosure, a significant loss of trust and disruption of the physician–patient relationship would occur.

USMLE-Style Questions

1. Two brothers have a rare inborn error of metabolism called carnitine-acylcarnitine translocase deficiency diagnosed in infancy. Their older sister is healthy. Their cells lack a mitochondrial enzyme. Which one of the following refutes the likelihood that an abnormal gene in the mother's mitochondrial DNA made the boys ill?

   A. Only girls can have a mitochondrially inherited disorder.
   B. Only oxidative phosphorylation reactions occur in the mitochondria.
   C. Symptoms should not have begun so soon after birth.
   D. The children's father is solely responsible.
   E. The two brothers had a healthy older sister.

The response options for items 2 to 5 are all the same, as follows. For each item in the set select the concept illustrated by the clinical situation.

   A. Allelic heterogeneity
   B. High carrier frequency
   C. New mutation
   D. Uniparental disomy
   E. Variable expressivity

2. A couple with normal vision from an isolated community have a child with autosomal recessive ornithine aminotransferase deficiency resulting in gyrate atrophy of the retina. The child grows up, marries a member of the same community who has normal vision, and has a child with the same enzyme deficiency.

3. A child has severe neurofibromatosis (NF1) with abnormal development of the sphenoid wing, dysplasia of the tibia, and optic nerve glioma. Her father is phenotypically normal; her mother seems clinically normal but has several large café-au-lait spots and areas of hypopigmentation, and slit-lamp examination shows that she has a few Lisch nodules (hamartomatous growths on the iris that are common in persons with NF1).

4. Parents of normal stature have a child with achondroplasia, the most common type of dwarfism, caused by a single mutation in one copy of the gene for fibroblast growth factor receptor type 3.

5. A patient with a recessive disorder is found to have inherited both copies of one chromosome from the same parent and no representative of that chromosome from the other parent.

SUGGESTED READINGS

Bomford A. Genetics of haemochromatosis. Lancet 2002;360:1673–1681.

Carey JC, Viskochil DH. Neurofibromatosis type 1: a model condition for the study of the molecular basis of variable expressivity in human disorders. Am J Med Genet 1999;89:7–13.

Bosma PJ, Chowdhury JR, Bakker C, et al. The genetic basis of the reduced expression of bilirubin UDP-glucuronosyltransferase 1 in Gilbert's syndrome. N Engl J Med 1995;333:1171–1175.

Schmid R. Gilbert's syndrome: a legitimate genetic anomaly? N Engl J Med 1995;333:1217–1218.

Kaplan M, Renbaum P, Levy-Lahad E, et al. Gilbert syndrome and glucose-6-phosphate dehydrogenase deficiency: a dose-dependent genetic interaction crucial to neonatal hyperbilirubinemia. Proc Natl Acad Sci USA 1997;94:12128–12132.

Ranum LPW, Day JW. Myotonic dystrophy: RNA pathogenesis comes into focus. Am J Hum Genet 2004; 793–804.

WEB RESOURCES

http://genetests.org
   Good reviews of myotonic dystrophy, 21-hydroxylase deficiency, Leber's hereditary optic neuropathy.

http://www.rarediseases.org/
   The National Organization for Rare Diseases (NORD) maintains an index of rare diseases and a listing of affiliated disease-oriented groups.

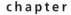

Cancer Genetics

Cancer refers to 100 or more diseases that all share the primary characteristic of uncontrolled cellular proliferation that may lead to a mass or tumor. It is the second leading cause of death in the United States behind heart disease. In 2003, about 1.3 million cases of cancer were diagnosed, and more than 1500 people died of cancer every day. The 5-year relative survival rate for individuals with cancer in the U.S. is 62%.

Cancer is a genetic disease resulting from a disruption of one or more genes. A minority of cancers (5–10%) are caused by inherited genetic mutations. Most cancers are caused by the cumulative effect of somatic genetic mutations over the life of an individual.

Cancers are characterized by the site of origin, the tissue type of origin, the degree of spread, and the molecular characteristics of the tumor. The tissue type is determined classically by microscopic appearance and molecular features such as cell surface receptors. Three principal types of cancer are described: sarcoma, carcinoma, and hematopoietic or lymphoid. **Sarcomas** arise from mesenchymal tissue, such as bone, muscle, and connective tissue. **Carcinomas** arise from epithelial tissue, such as skin and the linings of internal organs. **Hematopoietic** or **lymphoid cancers** arise from cells originating in the bone marrow.

GENES AND CANCER

Many genes have been implicated in the origin of cancer, or **carcinogenesis**:

- Genes in signaling pathways for cell proliferation
- Cytoskeletal components responsible for the maintenance of contact inhibition between cells
- Mitotic cycle regulators, programmed cell death processes
- Genes that detect and repair mutations occurring during the normal replication of DNA

Different types of genomic and genetic disruptions may lead to cancer. **Proto-oncogenes** are normally occurring genes responsible for cell growth and maturation. A gain-of-function mutation in a single allele of a proto-oncogene disrupts the normal feedback loops within a cell and causes uninterrupted cell growth—the cardinal feature of cancer. **Oncogenes** are mutated proto-oncogenes. **Tumor suppressor genes** are another type of cell cycle control gene that may require loss-of-function mutations of both alleles or a dominant negative mutation in one allele to cause abnormal cell growth. DNA repair genes suppress tumor growth as well. Chromosomal translocations may result in abnormal gene expression or the mixture of two genes (chimera) with a new function within the cell. Epigenetic changes may silence a gene (loss of function) and result in disruption of cellular growth control.

MULTISTEP EVOLUTION IN CANCER

All cancers start from a single cell. The cell typically develops a somatic mutation that increases the growth rate and gives it a competitive growth advantage over the neighboring cells. The daughter cells of the original cell, or **clones**, are genetically identical to the original and have the same proliferative advantage. A mutant clone could take over the organism given enough time, unlimited blood supply, and nutrients. A single mutation is rarely capable of providing the proliferative advantage needed for clones to progress to cancer, and other mutations are also necessary (Fig. 8.1). Each mutation adds a slight competitive advantage to its daughter cells until finally enough changes have occurred that the cells are capable of invading neighboring tissues, inducing growth of new blood vessels (angiogenesis), and spreading to distant sites in the body (metastasizing).

As the clones attempt to proliferate, the natural control mechanisms of the organism attempt to maintain normal growth. Most somatic mutations are repaired by normal DNA mechanisms. Cells that cannot be repaired usually activate apoptosis. Only those few cells that avoid repair and apoptosis are candidates for continued clonal proliferation.

CANCER RISK ASSESSMENT COUNSELING

Germline mutations in cell cycle control and DNA repair mechanisms result in hereditary cancer syndromes and a greatly increased risk of cancer. Only 5 to 10% of cancers are initiated by germline mutations (hereditary); the remainder are initiated by somatic mutations (sporadic). It is important that clinicians distinguish between hereditary and sporadic cancers so that they provide presymptomatic cancer risk assessment to families with a hereditary susceptibility. This assessment may result in recommendations for risk reduction or early detection, including changes in behavior (smoking cessation, weight loss, dietary changes), increased cancer screening (earlier initiation of and more frequent screening), genetic counseling, and genetic testing.

The family history is the most useful and cost-effective tool for differentiating between hereditary and sporadic cancers. A cancer family history should include at least three generations of family members, ethnicity or race, age at the time of diagnosis of cancer or at the time of death, cause of death, specific type and location of cancer, distinction

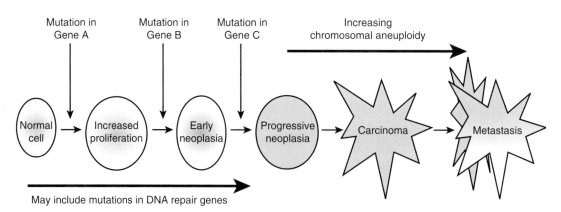

FIGURE 8.1 Multistep evolution in cancer. Each individual cancer and type of cancer may require varying numbers of mutations to progress to full-blown invasive cancer or carcinoma. (Adapted with permission from Fearon ER, Vogelstein B. A genetic model for colorectal tumorigenesis. Cell 1990;61:759.)

BOX 8.1

Family History Flags of a Hereditary Cancer Syndrome

- Cancer in two or more relatives
- Early age of diagnosis
- Multiple primary tumors
- Bilateral or multiple rare tumors

---

between site of origin (primary) and site of metastasis, and any precursor lesions or associated disorders.

All individuals with a personal history of cancer or a family history of cancer involving first- or second-degree relatives should have an assessment of their family medical information. A hereditary cancer syndrome may be suspected if any of the following factors are present: two or more relatives on the same side of the family with the same type of cancer, early age at diagnosis, several primary tumors, bilateral tumors or multiple rare cancers, a collection of cancers consistent with an inherited cancer syndrome, or evidence of autosomal dominant or recessive inheritance (Box 8.1).

If a hereditary cancer syndrome is suspected, genetic testing, assuming it is available, may be considered either through a Clinical Laboratories Improvement Act (CLIA) regulated clinical laboratory or through a research laboratory with subsequent CLIA laboratory confirmation. A listing of available tests may be found on http://genetests.org, a Web site supported by public funds. For maximum effectiveness and interpretation of results, the specific mutation must first be identified in a family. A living individual who has actually had the cancer of concern is needed and is frequently a different person from the family member expressing concern and desiring gene testing. Genetic testing of the affected person usually involves sequencing of the complete gene from leukocyte DNA, and the cost is proportional to the size of the gene (range: $300 to $3000). Once a mutation has been identified in the family, other as yet

unaffected family members may have gene testing to determine their cancer susceptibility. Gene testing for the family members may be targeted to the previously identified mutation for a cost of $250 to $350.

Genetic testing for adult-onset disorders should be performed only after appropriate counseling. Testing is not usually conducted on children younger than 18 years of age unless there is a risk of symptoms or disease in childhood. Presymptomatic gene tests have many far-reaching ramifications, including changes in health care management, psychological stresses, financial implications, and potential changes in family dynamics. At-risk individuals should be counseled about these ramifications in a nondirective manner before the health care professional obtains informed consent and draws a blood sample.

ONCOGENES

An oncogene is a normally occurring proto-oncogene in which a gain-of-function mutation has taken place (Box 8.2). Like other gain-of-function mutations, the oncogene results in a dominant phenotype within the cell; only one abnormal allele is necessary to change the normal cellular phenotype. A regulatory mutation may occur in a growth factor gene, resulting in increased expression or secretion of the product. A structural mutation may occur in growth factor receptors or signal transduction proteins that disable regulatory feedback mechanisms and allow autonomy of expression. Structural integrity of nuclear genes may be disrupted by chromosomal translocation, insertion of retroviral DNA, or gene amplification; all of these factors result in overexpression of the gene.

BOX 8.2

Functions of Proto-oncogenes
- Induce telomerase activity
- Block apoptosis
- Stimulate proliferation
- Increase blood supply

Oncogenes may also be activated by epigenetic mechanisms. Methylated CpG dinucleotides may develop a point mutation that prevents methylation, allowing a normally silenced gene to become active. Loss of normal imprinting may also allow both alleles to be expressed; the resulting extra dose of gene product acts as a gain-of-function.

Amplification

Amplification involves a multiplication of the number of copies of a gene, resulting in overexpression of the protein. Amplification may affect response to treatment and may be used to determine the appropriate management. Amplification is a somatic mutation and is considered one of the later steps in the evolution of cancer.

Clinical testing for amplification is used routinely in planning therapy for children with neuroblastoma, the most common malignant intra-abdominal tumor in children. The median age at diagnosis is 2 years. A neuroblastoma may originate from any sympathetic nervous system tissue, with the adrenal gland as the primary site in 38% of children and the abdomen, thorax, and neck as other common locations. There are at least three clinical patterns of neuroblastoma:

- Disease that is widespread at the time of diagnosis but that spontaneously regresses (stage 4S)
- Disease that is confined to the original location or nearby region (stages 1–3)
- Metastatic disease (stage 4), which frequently is lethal

Patients with neuroblastoma that is not metastatic are expected to survive with surgical treatment alone. Patients with stage 4 disease have an overall survival rate of 20% despite treatment protocols involving intensive multimodal therapeutic combinations. Some individuals diagnosed at stage 3 respond well to routine therapy, and some progress to stage 4. The challenge in the clinical management of patients with neuroblastoma is to identify cases in which less aggressive therapy can be safely used; fewer life-threatening side effects may occur as a result.

MYCN on 2p24.1 is amplified in 20 to 25% of primary neuroblastomas and is homologous to the *MYC* gene at 8p24. Amplification of *MYCN* without overexpression of the protein product predicts poor response to routine treatment for children diagnosed with neuroblastoma older than 1 year of age and is now considered an important part of clinical decision making.

Gene amplification occurs through mechanisms that may operate concurrently or sequentially and may be specific to the amplified gene. In neuroblastoma, for instance, methylation of the *CASP8* promoter region prevents expression of caspase-8 (cysteine protease with aspartic acid specificity) in the apoptotic cycle. The lack of apoptotic control may permit multiple copies of a normal *MYCN* gene to be created and inserted into the genomic DNA, frequently in locations other than its normal starting point on 2p24.1. Using fluorescent in situ hybridization (FISH), these insertions can be seen as **homogeneously staining regions** (HSRs) (Fig. 8.2—see color insert). Gene amplification may also occur in the form of small separate chromosomes, or **double minutes** (pronounced my-NOOTS). The gene copy number is greatly increased in both HSRs and double minutes. Comparative genomic hybridization may also be used to detect amplification (see Figure 3.6).

Amplification of the *HER2* gene with overexpression of the transmembrane tyrosine kinase occurs in 20 to 30% of breast cancers. Many of the known oncogenes encode aberrant protein tyrosine kinases and are associated with a significant number of human cancers. The epidermal growth factor receptor (EGFR) and HER2/neu are two transmembrane tyrosine kinases that are members of the erbB-signaling network. The *HER2/neu* proto-oncogene (also known as *c-erbB-2*) encodes a 185-kD transmembrane receptor with tyrosine kinase activity. Although it has no known ligand, it is activated by joining with other members of its protein family (EGFR, c-erbB-3, c-erbB-4) as heterodimers, usually through disulfide bonding between two cysteine amino acids. Receptor activation enhances tumor cell motility and protease secretion and invasion. It also modulates cell cycle checkpoint function, DNA repair, and apoptotic responses. This protein family may play an important role in normal mammary development. Patients with breast cancer who overexpress HER2/neu have a relatively unfavorable prognosis, short time before relapse of disease, and low survival rate.

Tissue-based detection methods of **immunohistochemistry** (IHC) or FISH are used to detect amplification through detection of overexpression of the protein product (Fig. 8.3—see color insert). IHC is less expensive and is easier to perform than FISH. However, it has a higher rate of false results due to variations in laboratory technique and in pathologist interpretation. FISH is a more costly, relatively difficult assay, yet it appears to be a better predictor of response to therapy and outcome.

Chromosomal Translocations

Human leukemias and lymphomas are typically caused by acquired chromosomal translocations that activate or create an oncogene. Chronic leukemias are characterized by normal differentiation of hematopoietic cells but increased proliferation. Acute leukemias are characterized by abnormalities in both differentiation and proliferation.

Acute myeloid leukemias (AML) have chromosomal translocations that most often result in loss-of-function changes to transcription factors required for normal hematopoietic development. These mutations alone, however, are not enough to cause AML. Activating mutations in hematopoietic tyrosine kinases may give a proliferative advantage to hematopoietic progenitor cells, and subsequent loss-of-function mutations in hematopoietic transcription factors may allow the conversion of chronic leukemia to acute leukemia.

Chronic myeloid leukemias (CML) are caused by gain-of-function activations of tyrosine kinases, such as Bcr/Abl, that confer a growth and survival advantage to hematopoietic progenitor cells but do not affect differentiation. CML is genetically characterized by the reciprocal translocation t(9;22)(q34;q11). The small derivative chromosome 22, the Philadelphia chromosome, was first described in 1960 and was for a long time the only genetic lesion consistently associated with human cancer.

The (9;22) translocation results in fusion of the 5' part of the *BCR* gene, normally located on chromosome 22, with the 3' part of the *ABL* gene on chromosome 9, giving origin to a *BCR/ABL* fusion gene, which is transcribed and then translated into a hybrid protein. The normal function of *BCR* is unknown. *ABL* encodes a tightly regulated tyrosine kinase whose normal function is unknown. The hybrid protein encodes a 210-kD protein with deregulated tyrosine kinase activity, which is highly expressed in CML cells. Scientists have described three main variants of *BCR/ABL*. All variants have a constant *ABL* portion and a variable length of the sequence of the *BCR* gene. These main variants are associated with distinct clinical types of human leukemias. Several other leukemias and lymphomas have been associated with chromosomal translocations (Table 8.1).

Hereditary Syndromes of Oncogenes

Oncogene mutations are usually somatic rather than germline. The two best known genes with germline mutations are *MET* and *RET*. *MET* encodes a transmembrane receptor for hepatocyte growth factor. However, a germline mutation in *MET* results in hereditary papillary renal carcinoma in families. The molecular biology of *RET* is discussed in Chapter 5. The RET receptor forms a dimer in the presence of its ligands. Germline gain-of-function mutations in *RET* are responsible for familial medullary thyroid carcinoma and multiple endocrine neoplasia (MEN) types 2A and 2B. Type 2A makes up 90% of cases of MEN2.

Individuals with MEN2A have an extremely high risk of medullary thyroid carcinoma (MTC), a tumor of the calcitonin-producing C cells of the thyroid, even before puberty. MTC must be treated surgically by thyroidectomy before the tumor extends through the capsule of the thyroid gland; current chemotherapy regimens are relatively ineffec-

TABLE 8.1 CHROMOSOMAL TRANSLOCATIONS ASSOCIATED WITH HEMATOPOIETIC MALIGNANCIES

CHROMOSOME REARRANGEMENT	GENES	LEUKEMIA, LYMPHOMA
t(9;22)(q34;q11)	p210 *BCR/ABL*	Chronic myeloid leukemia
t(9;22)(q34;q11)	p190 *BCR/ABL*	Acute lymphoblastic leukemia (Ph positive)
t(9;22)(q34;q11)	p230 *BCR/ABL*	Chronic neutrophilic leukemia (rarely)
dup 11q23	*MLL* duplication	Acute myeloid leukemia
t(8;21)(q22;q22)	*AML1/ETO*	Acute myeloid leukemia, M2 subtype[a]
t(8;14)(q24;q32)	*IgH/MYC*	Burkitt lymphoma
t(14;18)(q32;q21)	*IgH/BCL2*	Follicular lymphoma
t(2;5)(p23;q35)	*NPM-ALK*	Anaplastic large cell lymphoma

[a]Accounts for 15% of cases of acute myeloid leukemia.
Ph, Philadelphia chromosome.

tive against metastatic MTC. It is recommended that individuals at risk for MTC have a thyroidectomy before 5 years of age to prevent late diagnosis of MTC. Individuals in families affected by MEN2 are also at increased risk for pheochromocytoma, a tumor of sympathetic nervous tissue with excessive production of catecholamines, and for hyperparathyroidism, causing increased calcium levels and kidney stones. MEN2B is characterized by the features of MEN2A but has an earlier age of onset.

Historically, early detection of MTC was performed by stimulating the C cells with pentagastrin to cause increased production of calcitonin, measurable in the blood. The test was uncomfortable for patients because of severe nausea. In addition, sensitivity and specificity were not ideal. Prior to the availability of genetic testing, approximately 50% of at-risk individuals with normal calcitonin levels were found to have microscopic MTC at the time of thyroidectomy. Approximately 10% who were subsequently shown not to have the *RET* mutation developed elevated calcitonin levels, which resulted in unnecessary thyroidectomies. Gene testing for the *RET* mutation would have shown which individuals needed presymptomatic thyroidectomy with much more accuracy (Table 8.2). Testing for the *RET* gene is available clinically and should be considered for any individual with MTC.

TUMOR SUPPRESSOR GENES

Tumor suppressor genes are cell cycle control genes that contribute to abnormal cell growth when altered by a loss-of-function mutation of both alleles (Box 8.3). Most inherited cancer susceptibility syndromes are caused by

TABLE 8.2 LIKELIHOOD OF *RET* MUTATION IN FAMILIES WITH MEN2

PHENOTYPE	% *RET* MUTATION
MEN2A (MTC, pheochromocytoma, hyperparathyroidism)	
All 3 features	97
No hyperparathyroidism	99
No pheochromocytoma	100
MEN2B	95
Familial MTC	88
Other MTC	85
Total	92

Reprinted with permission from Eng C et al. The relationship between specific RET proto-oncogene mutations and disease phenotype in multiple endocrine neoplasia type 2. International RET mutation consortium analysis. JAMA 276:1575, 1996.
MEN2, Multiple endocrine neoplasia type 2; MTC, medullary thyroid carcinoma

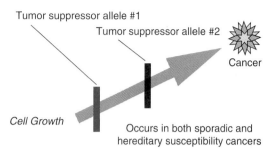

FIGURE 8.4 The two-hit theory of tumor suppressor gene inactivation, or Knudson hypothesis. Disruption of the first tumor suppressor allele may be inherited or acquired. Disruption of the second allele of the cell permits unchecked cell growth, resulting in a competitive growth advantage over neighboring cells and cancer.

---

germline mutations in these genes. Mutations may also be somatic. Gatekeeper genes have a rate-limiting function and regulate tumor growth through inhibition of growth or promotion of death. Caretaker genes prevent genetic instability and participate in DNA repair. If caretaker function is reduced, tumor formation is accelerated. Most inherited disorders associated with caretaker genes are discussed in Chapter 5.

Knudson Hypothesis

In 1971, well before the molecular techniques were available to support his theory, Alfred Knudson suggested that familial retinoblastoma is caused by an inherited inactivation of one allele of a tumor suppressor gene (the first hit). The phenotype within any cell would not be substantially altered because the other allele continues to function and produces a protein product. For the cellular phenotype to change, a second hit resulting in the loss of the second allele must be acquired somatically (Fig. 8.4). The cellular phenotype is recessive and requires the loss of both alleles. However, the observed inheritance pattern of the cancer phenotype is dominant, with variable penetrance, and age-related, gender-related, and environmental factors contributing to the variability.

It is now known that both cancers resulting from the inherited susceptibility produced by a germline mutation and sporadic cancers are caused by the two-hit hypothesis Knudson proposed. The difference is that individuals with an inherited susceptibility have a mutation in every cell in their body and need only a single sporadic mutation—a second hit—to initiate the development of cancer. An individual with an inherited cancer susceptibility mutation is relatively likely to have cancer at an earlier-than-expected age, to have it in more than one tissue or organ system, or to have a new occurrence of the same cancer. These features are characteristic of an inherited cancer susceptibility disorder.

An individual with no germline mutation may have an initial hit at any time but in only a few cells scattered throughout the body. A second hit is much less likely to occur in one of these previously affected cells because of simple probability. An individual who devel-

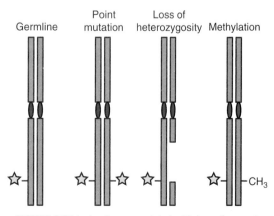

FIGURE 8.5 Mechanisms associated with loss of second allele. *Germline,* the normal initial heterozygosity of a person with an inherited mutation.

ops cancer in this manner is relatively likely to have cancer at an expected or older-than-expected age and is relatively unlikely to have more than one type of cancer or a new occurrence of the same cancer.

The second hit may occur in a number of ways: by point mutation, loss of heterozygosity (LOH), or epigenetic modification and gene silencing (Fig. 8.5). Regardless of the mechanism, the net effect is the loss of the normal allele. LOH is caused by a loss of genetic material from the normal chromosome, resulting in a mutated allele that is no longer opposed by a normally functioning allele. In some cases, the normal material is replaced by a duplication or crossing-over of material from the abnormal allele. It is also known now that even in retinoblastoma, the two-hit hypothesis is the starting point but is simplistic. Multiple genes may have to be altered to have tumor growth initiation, development, vascular supply, and spread.

Hereditary Syndromes of Tumor Suppressor Genes

Retinoblastoma

Retinoblastoma, an embryonic tumor of retinal cells that occurs in pre-school-aged children, is caused by abnormalities in the *RB1* gene on 13q14. This rare childhood cancer, which occurs in 1 in 17,000 live births, is historically important because of its role in the development of the Knudson hypothesis. The ability to treat this tumor successfully if the cancer is diagnosed early has resulted in the inclusion of an examination for retinoblastoma via the red reflex as a standard part of every infant and preschool child's pediatric examination. The red reflex is reflection of the normal red color of the retina through the pupil, as seen commonly in flash photography. Absence of the red reflex or the presence of a white reflex raises suspicion of an abnormality of the retina such as retinoblastoma, which may have replaced the normal red tissue.

Approximately 60% of retinoblastomas are sporadic, resulting in only one tumor in one eye, and the average age of onset is 24 to 30 months. The remaining 40% are caused by an inherited mutation in *RB1* that results in unilateral, multifocal, or bilateral tumors, and the average age of onset is 12 months. Individuals with familial retinoblastoma have an increased risk of osteosarcomas or fibrosarcomas and melanomas in later life. Genetic counseling should be offered to all members of families with a history of retinoblastoma, and genetic testing of affected individuals should be considered.

Somatic loss of the retinoblastoma protein (Rb) function has also been associated with many cancers. *RB1*, considered a gatekeeper gene, encodes for a phosphoprotein active in cell cycle control. Rb is primarily controlled through phosphorylation by cyclin-dependent kinases (CDKs). In the hypophosphorylated state, Rb actively binds to and inhibits the E2F transcription factor that regulates the transcription of many genes required in S-phase. Because Rb is progressively phosphorylated by cyclin–CDK complexes in the G1 phase, it eventually is inactivated and releases the E2F transcription factor, allowing E2F to function and the cell to enter the S phase. Elements of the Rb regulatory pathway may be somatically mutated in almost 100% of human tumors, sometimes by recessive loss-of-function mutations (Rb) and sometimes by dominant gain-of-function mutations (cyclin).

Familial Adenomatous Polyposis

Familial adenomatous polyposis (FAP) is an inherited syndrome of predisposition to colorectal cancer in which hundreds to thousands of precancerous colonic polyps develop, usually beginning in adolescence (Fig. 8.6). FAP occurs in approximately 1 in 10,000 individuals. Without colectomy, the risk of colon cancer is almost 100%, and the average age at discovery of cancer is 39 years. Diseases that may occur outside the colon include polyps of the stomach and duodenum; bone tumors or cysts (osteomas); abnormalities of the teeth, such as too many teeth or teeth present at birth; congenital hypertrophy of the retina pigment epithelium; epidermoid cysts; and desmoid tumors (benign soft tissue sarcomas originating from tendons and ligaments). Cancers may rarely form in these other benign growths.

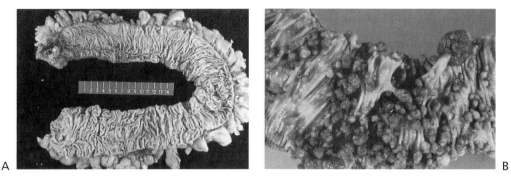

FIGURE 8.6 A. Normal colon mucosa demonstrated in surgical specimen that has been opened to expose the interior of the colon. **B.** Interior surface of a colon from a person with familial adenomatous polyposis who has hundreds of adenomatous polyps. (Courtesy of Dr. C. Hitchcock, Ohio State University Department of Pathology.)

Rarely, an individual with FAP may develop a medulloblastoma of the brain, or Turcot (pronounced ter-KOH) syndrome.

FAP is caused by a germline mutation in the adenomatous polyposis coli (*APC*) gene on 5q21–22. APC normally has at least two principal duties within the cell: (*a*) binding intracytoplasmic β-catenin, a transcription activator, and promoting its degradation (a gatekeeper function) (Fig. 8.7), and (*b*) responsibility for microtubule assembly at the kinetochore of chromosomes (a caretaker function). Mutations in *APC* follow the Knudson hypothesis. *APC* mutations, whether germline or somatic, are believed to be needed to initiate the sequence for the development of any colorectal adenomatous polyp, the first step in the development of most colorectal cancers (Fig. 8.1). Abnormal APC protein releases β-catenin, allowing the β-catenin to move to the

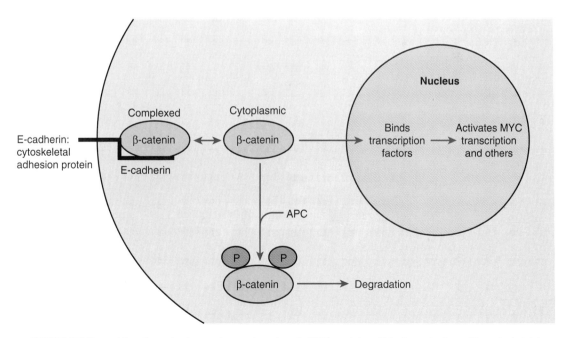

FIGURE 8.7 Normal function of adenomatous polyposis coli (APC) protein within the cytoplasm. The cytoskeletal adhesion protein E-cadherin complexes with β-catenin. Free cytoplasmic β-catenin is bound by APC, phosphorylated, and targeted for degradation. Unbound β-catenin enters the nucleus and participates in the transcription of nuclear genes.

nucleus, where it becomes part of a multiprotein transcription factor complex that increases cellular proliferation. Acquired mutations in the 3′ portion of the gene result in abnormal microtubule assembly, producing chromosomal instability and the tendency for increasingly abnormal chromosomal configurations within a tumor cell. These 3′ mutations tend to occur late in the multistep evolution of cancer.

Inherited abnormalities in the *APC* gene are associated with several interrelated phenotypes (Fig. 8.8). Attenuated polyposis correlates with mutations in the extreme 5′ portion of the gene. Polyps are relatively few (<100), the age of onset of polyps is relatively late (mid 40s), and there is a predilection for the right side of the colon. Gardner syndrome describes individuals with classical colonic features of FAP with dental abnormalities and skin lesions. An autosomal dominant desmoid tumor syndrome has been described with *APC* mutations in classical FAP but without the classical colonic features. Individuals who have more than 15 adenomatous polyps should receive genetic counseling and should consider genetic testing.

Hereditary Nonpolyposis Colorectal Cancer Syndrome

Hereditary nonpolyposis colorectal cancer syndrome (HNPCC) is caused by an abnormality in the mismatch DNA repair system (see Chapter 5). Allelic heterogeneity is

the rule; defects in the *MLH1, MSH2, MSH6, PMS1,* and *PMS2* genes all result in the HNPCC phenotype, with some minor phenotypic variations. Mutations in *MLH1* and *MSH2* are by far the most common causes of HNPCC.

HNPCC is the most common known cause of inherited colorectal cancer, accounting for 2 to 5% of all cases. Individuals with HNPCC are likely to develop cancer fairly young (<45 years). An individual with a germline mutation has up to an 85% risk of developing colorectal cancer, compared with a 6% risk in a normal individual. In HNPCC, unlike in sporadic colorectal cancer, colorectal cancer occurs more commonly on the right or proximal side of the colon. HNPCC is also likely to occur simultaneously in more than one location in the colon (synchronous) and is also likely to have a second primary occurrence at a later time (metachronous). Affected women have a 40 to 60% risk of endometrial cancer. Other malignancies may also occur in the ovary, stomach, urinary tract (particularly transitional cell cancers), small bowel, bile ducts, and sebaceous glands. Rarely, an individual with HNPCC may develop a glioblastoma of the brain, a syndrome given the same eponymic designation as a person affected with FAP and a brain tumor, or Turcot syndrome.

Colon polyps occur in HNPCC, although at a much lower frequency than in FAP (dozens

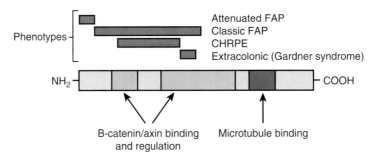

FIGURE 8.8 Germline mutations in specific regions of the adenomatous polyposis coli (*APC*) gene are associated with specific phenotypes and subsets of the features of familial adenomatous polyposis (FAP). *Gray bars*, the region of the APC gene in which germline mutations may be found associated with the stated phenotype. Note the lack of germline mutations in the carboxy terminal. Second-hit somatic mutations may occur anywhere. CHRPE, congenital hypertrophy of the retina pigment epithelium. (Adapted with permission from Kinzler KW, Vogelstein B. Lessons from hereditary colorectal cancer. Cell 1996;87:159; and Fodde R. APC, signal transduction and genetic instability in colorectal cancer. Nat Rev Cancer 2001;1:55.)

rather than hundreds). Annual colonoscopy has been shown to reduce the rate of cancer occurrence in HNPCC, likely through the removal of polyps before progression to cancer, as well as permitting cancer diagnosis at an earlier and more treatable stage.

Because of the allelic heterogeneity, clinical criteria are used to screen families for HNPCC. The Amsterdam II criteria stipulate that an individual must have three or more relatives with an HNPCC-associated tumor (colorectal, endometrial, small bowel, ureter, or renal pelvis). Two generations must be involved, and one of the affected relatives must be a first-degree relative of the other two. In addition, one or more individuals must have been diagnosed with cancer before 50 years of age. The Amsterdam II criteria do not detect everyone with an HNPCC genetic mutation, however, and other screening methods have been developed.

The mismatch repair mechanism finds and corrects slippages in microsatellite DNA regions, which are present in several genes associated with carcinogenesis in the colon. The *APC* gene has several microsatellite regions. Lack of mismatch repair of these *APC* microsatellites is consistent with the occasional initiation of polyp formation in individuals affected with HNPCC. A defective repair mechanism allows variability in normally occurring microsatellite repeat regions (microsatellite instability, or MSI), which can be detected by studying tumor tissue, even after treatment with formalin. MSI may be seen in 10 to 15% of sporadic colorectal cancers, 20 to 30% of sporadic endometrial cancers, and 95% of cancer types associated with HNPCC. MSI is a reasonable screening method for any colorectal or endometrial cancer, particularly for individuals with a family history of HNPCC-associated cancers or who are younger than 50 years. MSI assays are available in many clinical laboratories (Fig. 8.9).

The occurrence of MSI in sporadic colorectal and endometrial cancers is associated with epigenetic modification of one of the mismatch repair genes, usually *MLH1*. Methylation of the promoter region of *MLH1* may be one of the steps in the evolution of cancer. Analysis of

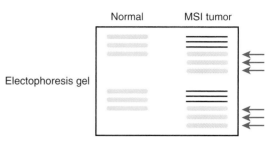

FIGURE 8.9 Gel electrophoresis demonstrating a normal control and a colorectal tumor sample with microsatellite instability (MSI). Arrows, bands with added bases in variable numbers. Radioisotope-labeled probes are used in the laboratory and x-ray film used to capture the release of radiation (autoradiograph) and the ladder rung pattern. The resulting pattern may be seen as a smear rather than discrete bands.

methylation should be done in an MSI-positive tumor; if it is present, the cancer can be considered sporadic. If methylation is absent, genetic counseling should be provided, and mismatch repair gene testing should be considered.

Other genes involved in carcinogenesis have microsatellite regions and may be affected by defects in the mismatch repair mechanism. Transforming growth factor (TGF) β is a multifunctional cytokine. One of its many functions is to serve as a cellular growth inhibitor. Cancer can develop when any portion of the TGFβ signaling pathway is altered (Fig. 8.10). The extracellular TGFβ binds to the TGFβ receptor that consists of two proteins (TGFβRI and TGFβRII), which are serine kinases. The TGFβRII kinase phosphorylates the TGFβRI kinase, activating it. The entire receptor complex then phosphorylates cytoplasmic SMAD proteins that translocate into the nucleus and act in cooperation with other transcription factors to induce specific genes. SMAD proteins are encoded by MADH genes (named for the homology with the Mad cytoplasmic proteins found in *Drosophila*). Mutations in the nuclear target genes, *MADHs*, or TGFβ receptors are all associated with human benign tumor formation or cancers. TGFβRII has a microsatellite of 10 adenosine residues in the region that codes for the cysteine-rich extracellular area of the protein. Lack of mismatch repair of this mi-

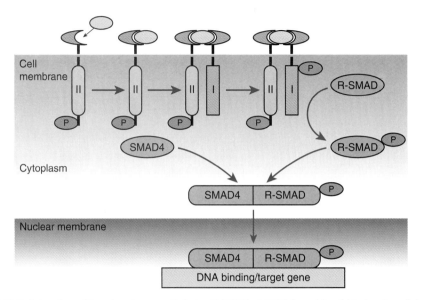

FIGURE 8.10 Cell signaling of transforming growth factor-β (TGFβ). A TGFβ ligand (*oval*) binds extracellularly to type II TGFβ receptor. On hetero-oligomerization with a type I TGFβ receptor, the type I receptor is transphosphorylated and activated. The activated complex phosphorylates receptor-regulated SMADs (R-SMADs) then associate with the common SMAD (SMAD4). The R-SMAD:SMAD4 complex translocates to the nucleus, where it regulates DNA transcription. (Adapted with permission from Waite KA, Eng C. From developmental disorder to heritable cancer: it's all in the BMP/TGF-beta family. Nat Rev Genet 2003;4:763.)

crosatellite region alters the TGFβRII protein transmission through the signal cascade and promotes cell growth. Sporadic somatic mutations in non-MSI tumors have also been found in the intracellular kinase regions of the TGFβ receptors and in SMAD proteins.

Hereditary Breast/Ovarian Cancer Syndrome

Breast cancer is also an important component of several inherited cancer susceptibility syndromes, including Li-Fraumeni syndrome (*TP53* gene), Cowden syndrome (*PTEN* gene), and hereditary breast/ovarian cancer syndrome.

Hereditary breast/ovarian cancer syndrome is thought to account for 5% of cases of breast cancer and is caused by germline mutations in either the *BRCA1* or *BRCA2* gene. (The name BRCA is derived from *breast cancer*.) Several clinical and familial features indicate an increased likelihood of a mutation in *BRCA1* or *BRCA2*, including multiple cases of premenopausal or early-onset breast cancer in the family, ovarian can-

cer with a family history of breast or ovarian cancer, cancer of the breast and ovary in the same woman, bilateral or multifocal primary breast cancers, Ashkenazi Jewish heritage, and male breast cancer.

It is important to assess both the maternal and paternal family histories. The father's medical history may not contribute to the assessment because of gender effects on gene penetrance, but he may still transmit the genetic mutation. Validated risk assessment software is available to calculate the likelihood of a *BRCA1* or *BRCA2* mutation based on clinical and family histories (http://astor.som.jhmi.edu/brcapro/).

Knowledge of ethnic origin is essential to assist in testing and interpretation of findings. Any individual of Ashkenazi Jewish heritage has a 2 to 3% risk of having one of three founder mutations in either *BRCA1* (187delAG, 5382insC) or *BRCA2* (6174delT). The mutations are also seen in non-Jewish Eastern Europeans. Iceland, which is home to a geographically isolated founder population, has a 2.5% occurrence of the 999del5 *BRCA2* mutation in its population. African Americans, on the other hand, have a 50 to 55% likelihood of variants in the genetic sequence that have yet to be classified as either a polymorphism or a missense mutation.

Women who have a germline mutation in *BRCA1* or *BRCA2* have a 40 to 85% lifetime risk of breast cancer and a 10 to 40% lifetime risk of ovarian cancer. (Women in the general population have an 11% lifetime risk of breast cancer and a 1.5% risk of ovarian cancer.) The specific risks of developing other types of cancer demonstrate locus and allelic heterogeneity. *BRCA1* mutations are associated with higher risks of breast and ovarian cancer in women and increased prostate cancer risks in men. Mutations in certain regions of the *BRCA1* gene are associated with the highest risks of ovarian cancer. Mutations in *BRCA2* are associated with lower risks of breast and ovarian cancer but increased risk of other cancers (pancreas and thyroid). Men with *BRCA2* mutations have an increased risk of developing breast cancer.

Identification of a *BRCA1* or *BRCA2* mutation in a family permits presymptomatic identification of at-risk individuals and initiation of enhanced health management procedures. Recommendations for at-risk women include initiation of mammography at 25 years of age rather than at 40 and twice-yearly ovarian screening with transvaginal ultrasonography and CA-125 tumor marker levels. Surgical removal of the ovaries before 40 to 45 years of age is recommended, and prophylactic mastectomies may be an option for some women. Although surgical approaches reduce the cancer risk by 90 to 95%, some risk remains because of residual breast tissue, particularly if the nipple and areola are not removed, and the common embryonic origin of peritoneal and ovarian tissue, which may be associated with primary peritoneal cancer.

BRCA1 and *BRCA2* are part of the BRCA1-associated genome surveillance complex mechanism that repairs single-stranded breaks, double-stranded breaks, or cross-links in the DNA caused either during the normal replication process or by chemical agents or ionizing radiation (see Chapter 5, Figure 5.13). The exact mechanisms of action are under investigation.

ETHICS | Adenomatous Polyposis Coli Testing: When Technical Ability Outpaces the Physician's Knowledge

Francis Giardiello and colleagues from Johns Hopkins University published "The Use and Interpretation of Commercial *APC* Gene Testing for Familial Adenomatous Polyposis" in the March 20, 1997, edition of the New England Journal of Medicine (336:823–827). The investigators conducted a telephone interview of all physicians who had ordered adenomatous polyposis coli (*APC*) gene tests from a commercial laboratory. In the interview, the investigators asked about the following issues:

- Indications for conducting gene testing
- Whether genetic counseling had been given
- Whether written informed consent was obtained
- Physicians' understanding of the significance of the test results

Sequencing of the entire gene was not commonly performed at the time of the study. The assay was capable of detecting only mutations that resulted in a truncated protein, and it detected mutations in only 70 to 80% of families with clinical features of FAP. Results were reported as "positive" if protein truncation occurred, as "no mu-

(continues)

tation found" if no mutation had yet been identified in the family, and as "negative" when no mutation was found in a member of a family in which a mutation had previously been detected.

Some patients had clinical features of FAP, and others were presymptomatic. Although the test was ordered as indicated in 83% of cases, adherence to other testing standards was less strict. Only 19% of the patients received genetic counseling before testing, and only 17% provided written informed consent. About 20% of the presymptomatic patients had testing before the *APC* mutation was identified in an affected family member. Almost 32% of patients received an incorrect interpretation of the test from their physician, based on errors in the physicians' understanding of the test. These physicians did not consider the limitations of the test assay and its effect on the detection of mutations, so they did not report the difference between a result of "negative" and "no mutation found" to their patients. A "negative" result would clear the patient of the risk of FAP and the need for increased cancer screening. A "no mutation found" result should not have been used to reduce cancer screening, because the family could fall within the 20 to 30% of FAP caused by nontruncating mutations.

Gene testing is very different from most medical laboratory studies. A routine chemistry profile or complete blood count provides numerical results with known ranges. The accuracy of gene testing varies from gene to gene depending on the proportion of mutations associated with intragenic sequence changes, deletions or duplications of segments of DNA, or extragenic changes in promoter or control regions. The assay used to conduct the test is accurate only in detecting the changes it is capable of detecting. For example, gene sequencing is extremely accurate in the detection of intragenic sequence changes but does not detect deletion of an entire exon or any changes outside the boundaries of the probes used to initiate the sequencing reaction.

The ethical principle of **informed consent** requires the practitioner to provide appropriate information to the patient about the procedure or test he or she is about to undergo. Patients cannot adequately consent if neither they nor the practitioner understand the benefits, risks, and limitations of what is about to occur. It is the responsibility of the ordering physician to know the uses and limitations of a diagnostic test and to be able to interpret the test results appropriately for the patient. Health care providers must be lifelong learners and keep themselves informed about new diagnostic and therapeutic aids. Practitioners must also recognize their own limitations and be prepared to refer patients to others with the appropriate knowledge and specialization.

USMLE-Style Questions

The following questions refer to this pedigree:

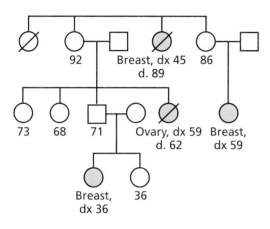

1. Which of the following genes is most likely to be abnormal in the family?
    a. *BCR, ABL*
    b. *BRCA1, BRCA2*
    c. *MLH1, MSH2*
    d. *RET, MET*
    e. *TP53, PTEN*

2. Individual II-3 does not express the phenotype. Which of the following is the most likely explanation?
    a. Adoption or nonpaternity of III-1
    b. Germline mosaicism in I-2
    c. Maternal imprinting in I-2 and I-5
    d. Nonpenetrance because of gender effects
    e. Unaffected parents prevented transmission

3. Individual III-2 is concerned about her risk of developing breast or ovarian cancer and desires gene testing. Her complete family history was taken. Her mother has a sister who had breast cancer diagnosed at age 42. Which of the following is the most appropriate person in the family to test initially?
    a. I-2
    b. II-3

    c. II-6
    d. III-1
    e. III-2

4. The ethnic background of the family is not shown in the pedigree. Given the family history, which of the following ethnic backgrounds would raise the most concern of a cancer susceptibility syndrome?
    a. African American
    b. Appalachian
    c. Ashkenazi Jewish
    d. British
    e. Lutheran

SUGGESTED READINGS

Knudson AG. Cancer genetics. Am J Med Genet 2002; 11:96–102.

Venkitaraman AR. A growing network of cancer susceptibility genes. N Engl J Med 2003;348:1917–1919.

Lynch HT, de la Chapelle A. Hereditary colorectal cancer. N Engl J Med 2003;348:919–932.

Chung DC, Rustgi AK. The hereditary nonpolyposis colorectal cancer syndrome: genetics and clinical implications. Ann Intern Med 2003;138:560–570.

Wooster R, Weber, BL. Breast and ovarian cancer. N Engl J Med 2003;348:2339–2347.

Olopade OI, Fackenthal JD, Dunston G, et al. Breast cancer genetics in African Americans. Cancer 2003;97(1 Suppl):236–245.

Giardiello FM, Brensinger JD, Petersen GM, et al. The use and interpretation of commercial *APC* gene testing for familial adenomatous polyposis. N Engl J Med 1997;336:823–827.

Veatch RM. Consent, confidentiality, and research. N Engl J Med 1997;336:869–870.

WEB RESOURCES

http://cancer.gov/
    National Cancer Institute. Contains information about the treatment of different cancer types for patients and health care professionals. The cancer genetics section may be found at http://www.nci.nih.gov/cancerinfo/prevention-genetics-causes/genetics.

http://clinicaltrials.gov
    National Institutes of Health. Linking patients to medical research.

http://genetests.org
    GeneTests. Listing of clinical and research laboratories offering testing for various hereditary cancer syndromes.

Complex Diseases

The genetics of cancer are not completely understood, but the study of it is the first successful step in our knowledge of the genetics of complex diseases—the nonmendelian disorders that occur in families more frequently than permitted by chance alone but that show no clear classical inheritance pattern. These complex diseases, among the most common diseases encountered by medical practitioners, include coronary artery disease, congestive heart failure, hypertension, stroke, diabetes, autoimmune disorders, Parkinson disease, psychiatric and psychological disorders, and commonly encountered birth defects. A host of other disorders and common physical traits are also considered to be inherited in a complex manner.

Since the 1980s, the tools and infrastructure provided by the Human Genome Project have permitted the most rapid influx of biomedical discoveries in recorded history. The discovery and identification of genes responsible for single-gene disorders has increased tremendously. However, the genes that have been identified are primarily relatively rare alleles with large phenotypic effects. Scientific research is just beginning to contribute to our knowledge of the following:

- Common alleles that have small to moderate effects
- Genes that have a far greater phenotypic impact when combined than they do separately (**polygenic** or **multigenic traits,** which may be caused by **modifier genes**)
- Interactions among genes, epigenetic factors, and the microenvironment of the cell
- Interactions between germline genes and environmental factors outside the individual

Human disease results from a spectrum of causative agents. Diseases may be caused by mendelian traits with almost 100% penetrance, dominant traits with incomplete penetrance, polygenic or multigenic disorders, multifactorial disorders with extensive environmental effects, or almost 100% environmental factors.

No single-gene disorder produces a phenotype that is completely independent of other genetic, environmental, or developmental factors. Trauma victims may have genetic components to injury response and wound healing. They may even have genes that contribute to a willingness to engage in risk-seeking behavior. In addition, infectious diseases are influenced by a person's genetic susceptibility to the infectious organism and activity of drug-metabolizing enzymes.

Determination of the various influences on disease phenotypes in a complex biological system is one of the objectives of medical research in the upcoming decades. The task is difficult because of the need to have the exact confluence of factors to produce a given phe-

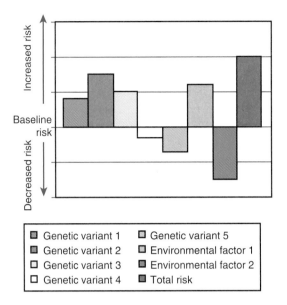

Genetic variant 1   Genetic variant 5
Genetic variant 2   Environmental factor 1
Genetic variant 3   Environmental factor 2
Genetic variant 4   Total risk

FIGURE 9.1 A variety of genetic and environmental factors may contribute to the disease or trait phenotype through either an increase or a decrease in risk. Each phenotype has its own unique mix of contributing factors. Phenotypes with one or two predominant factors are more easily studied than those with several equivalent factors.

notype, including factors that may protect against disease and some that may enhance susceptibility (Fig. 9.1).

THRESHOLD MODEL

The theoretical models of polygenic traits assume that all individuals have a susceptibili-ty to develop the trait but that a threshold must be reached before the trait is expressed (Fig. 9.2). Individuals from families who have already demonstrated the trait are assumed to be at greater risk for the trait than the gener-al population. The normal distribution curve for this group is farther to the right along the risk axis. The threshold level is fixed for the

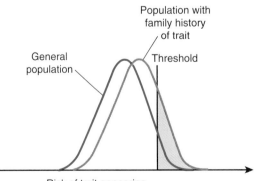

FIGURE 9.2 Any normally distributed population has a risk of having a trait appear. Those in the population whose risk is above a certain threshold demonstrate the phenotype (shaded area). Increasing values on the x-axis represent increasing risk. The population that has already demonstrated an individual with the trait has a relative susceptibili-ty, which is shifted to the right. More individuals in this group will have the trait than will the general population.

particular trait, but the recurrence risk is greater in members of these at-risk families because of the increase in susceptibility. As more affected individuals are reported in the family, the susceptibility curve is assumed to shift even more to the right, and the risk of recurrence climbs proportionately. These disorders exhibit a **familial** tendency in which the trait does not appear to have a mendelian single-gene pattern but occurs more often than is accounted for by chance.

In many isolated birth defects, including congenital heart disease, spina bifida, and cleft lip with or without cleft palate, if a single first-degree relative is affected, the recurrence risk is 3 to 5%. If two first-degree relatives are affected, the risk roughly doubles (~10%). If three first-degree relatives are affected, the risk may double again (~20%). If both parents and one or more siblings are affected, the risk may approach that of an autosomal dominant disorder (40–45%).

In adult-onset complex disorders, the recurrence risk is somewhat lower. For example, sporadic cancers have an approximate recurrence risk in first-degree relatives equal to approximately twice the risk in the general population. If a woman in the general population has a 1.5% risk of developing ovarian cancer at some time in her life, the daughter or sister of a woman with ovarian cancer has about a 3% risk of developing ovarian cancer.

MODIFIER GENES

Modifier genes are not associated with disease origin, but once disease susceptibility is present or the disease has developed, these genes modify the severity of phenotypic expression of the disease. Only a few specific modifier genes have been recognized; the identification of others is inevitable.

A modifier gene plays a role in idiopathic chronic pancreatitis, the leading cause of non-alcoholic chronic pancreatitis. Approximately 10 to 40% of individuals with idiopathic chronic pancreatitis have two mutations in their *CFTR* genes but have not been diagnosed with cystic fibrosis (see Chapter 6), a disease

known to produce pancreatic duct abnormalities along with respiratory symptoms. About 5 to 20% of individuals with idiopathic chronic pancreatitis also have a missense mutation (N34S) in one of their *SPINK1* genes on 5q32. Normally, the *SPINK1* gene encodes for a serine protease inhibitor that prevents activation of the pancreatic digestive enzymes prior to their entry into the duodenum. Activation prior to the gut is predicted to damage the pancreas through autodigestion. In one study, the risk of pancreatitis was increased 14-fold in individuals heterozygous for the N34S mutation on *SPINK1*, 40-fold in individuals homozygous for mutations in *CFTR*, and 600-fold in individuals with both mutations. *SPINK1* alone is a low-penetrant susceptibility gene for pancreatitis, but in combination with *CFTR*, it is a significant modifier gene for *CFTR*-induced pancreatitis.

Another established example of a modifier gene is melanocortin-1 receptor gene (*MC1R*) on 16q24.3, which plays a role in the development of the skin cancer melanoma. The skin and hair normally produce two types of melanin, the red pheomelanin and the black eumelanin. Eumelanin protects against damage from the sun's ultraviolet (UV) radiation, and pheomelanin may increase UV-induced skin damage by its tendency to release free radicals in response to UV radiation. Individuals with red hair and fair skin primarily produce pheomelanin, fail to tan, and have freckles. They are also at risk for melanoma caused by UV radiation. The relative proportions of the two types of melanin are regulated by melanocyte-stimulating hormone, which acts on melanocytes through the melanocortin-1 receptor to increase the synthesis of eumelanin. Some MC1R variants have a reduced ability to initiate cyclic adenosine monophosphate (cAMP) stimulation. People who are homozygous for these variants have red hair and fair skin. However, some people who may be heterozygotes or compound heterozygotes have red hair. Differences in the type of red hair color depending on the genotype have been reported. Other persons who are heterozygous for *MC1R* have dark hair but fair skin, freckles, and difficulty tanning.

Inability to tan has long been associated with an increased risk (~100-fold) of cutaneous melanoma. (Cutaneous melanoma appears to develop through a separate molecular pathway from ocular melanoma.) Approximately 60% of the population of Australia is thought to be heterozygous for *MC1R* variants. Melanoma is a major public health concern in Australia, which has high exposure to UV radiation.

The gene for cyclin-dependent kinase inhibitor-2A (*CDKN2A*) on 9p21, which has also been referred to as p16 or $p16^{INK4}$, normally induces cell cycle arrest in G1 by inhibiting the phosphorylation of the Rb protein by the cyclin-dependent kinases CDK4 and CDK6. Individuals who are heterozygous for germline loss-of-function mutations of *CDKN2A* have an increased risk of cutaneous melanoma (50%) along with an increased susceptibility to pancreatic cancer. Individuals who are heterozygous for mutations in both *CDKN2A* and *MC1R* have an 85% risk of melanoma that appears not to be accounted for solely by the fair skin associated with MC1R variants. *MC1R* is therefore considered to be both a low-penetrance melanoma gene and a modifier gene of *CDKN2A*.

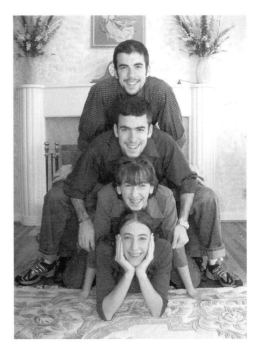

FIGURE 9.3 Four siblings consisting of two sets of monozygotic twins, 20 and 15 years of age, confirmed by DNA polymorphisms. Even though the genetically determined facial features are very similar, environmental factors, such as hairstyle and clothing, contribute to the appearance of each as a unique individual. (Courtesy of D. Westman, Columbus, Ohio.)

TOOLS FOR STUDY OF COMPLEX DISEASES

Twin Studies

It can be very difficult to determine the relative contribution of genes and environment to the development of complex diseases. Individuals with shared genes (i.e., a biological family) usually share a similar environment as well. Because of their genetic relationships and the similarities in intrauterine and early childhood environments, twin studies have provided insight into the relative contribution of genes and later environment on the development of complex diseases.

Monozygotic (MZ), or identical, twins have alleles in common at every locus; they originate from a single fertilized egg and separate into two embryos within the first 2 weeks of life. However, just like any other individuals, they acquire mutations in alleles

with time and age. MZ twins always are the same gender (Fig. 9.3). The intrauterine environment is similar; 70 to 75% share the placenta, although only 1 to 2% actually share the amniotic sac. In addition, early childhood environments are similar for MZ twins.

Dizygotic (DZ), or fraternal, twins are no more alike genetically than any two siblings; they originate from two separate ova and two separate sperm. However, unlike siblings and other first-degree relatives, they share the intrauterine environment and have similar early childhood environments. Because one-third of DZ twins are male-female pairs, gender influences may be present.

If both individuals in a pair of twins are affected with a disease, they are **concordant.** Diseases that are caused solely by inherited genes would be expected to have a 100% concordance in MZ twins. Diseases that are more often concordant in MZ twins than in DZ twins are thought to have a stronger genetic component than an environmental component.

Linkage Studies

Linkage is used to study complex diseases in individuals and families. When a disease is concordant in first-degree relatives (siblings, parent, and child), genetic studies may be performed to determine whether a genetic locus can be **linked** to the phenotype. Historically, large families with many affected individuals have been used to discover genes that cause highly penetrant single-gene disorders. Some genes have been discovered by study of one or two extended families. Complex diseases are less concordant in family members than mendelian disorders and are more likely to be caused by a combination of genetic polymorphisms, resulting in subtle changes in the interaction of a number of genes or the gene expression levels. Concordance in smaller family groups may be used, but many more family groups are needed (i.e., hundreds of affected sibling pairs or parent–child trios).

Siblings affected with the same complex disease are likely to share the same chromosomal region that carries the disease locus. Because any single pair of siblings shares 25% of their DNA, the study of multiple affected sibling pairs is necessary to pinpoint regions of DNA that are associated with a complex disease. If multiple alleles influence the disease, multiple regions can be expected to be linked to the phenotype. Multiple densely spaced markers (**multipoint linkage**) are used across the genome to enhance the likelihood of finding DNA regions that are identical by descent (truly inherited) rather than identical by chance.

Association Studies

When two alleles or phenotypes occur together in a population in a nonrandom manner with statistical significance, they are **associated.** Statistical association of an allele with a phenotype does not prove that one causes the other but only that further studies are necessary. More than 95% of studies that found associations between two entities have never been substantiated by other investigators, so to avoid biased results, care must be taken in selecting the appropriate population. Alleles for disease susceptibility that contribute to complex diseases may also be sought in population association studies. Alleles that confer only weak susceptibility may be more easily found through association studies than linkage studies. Microarray analysis of single-nucleotide polymorphisms may serve as a more rapid screen for associations. Founder populations with relatively little diversity in their DNA (e.g., Finnish, Icelandic, Amish peoples) may also assist in the initial assessment of association, and studies of more heterogeneous multiethnic populations should follow to confirm the association in a broader group.

The level of association may be quantified by the **relative risk,** an epidemiological measure used to quantify the association between either a susceptibility gene or an environmental agent and a disease phenotype. The relative risk is the ratio of incidence of disease in exposed individuals to the incidence of disease in unexposed individuals. If a disease is equally likely in people with or without a specific allele or genotype, the relative risk equals 1.0. A relative risk of 10 indicates that a person with the susceptibility gene has a 10 times as much risk of disease as the rest of the population.

CONGENITAL COMPLEX DISEASES

Hirschsprung Disease

Hirschsprung disease (**HSCR**), or congenital intestinal aganglionosis, is caused by absence of the nerve cells normally present in the wall of the large bowel and required for normal peristalsis. Abdominal distention results from inability to have a bowel movement (Fig. 9.4). The absence of the nerve cells is due to a failure of neural crest–derived intestinal ganglion cells to migrate into the intestinal tract at the appropriate time during embryological development. HSCR occurs in 1 in 5000 newborn infants. Inheritance does not usually appear to be mendelian. The recurrence risk to siblings is about 3 to 4%, which is characteristic of a multifactorial disorder.

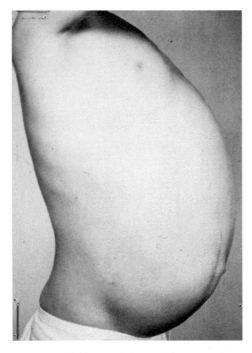

FIGURE 9.4 Child with abdominal distention due to colonic distention from the aganglionosis in Hirschsprung disease. (Reprinted with permission from Passage E. Dissecting Hirschsprung Disease, Nature Genetics 2002; 1:11–12. Courtesy of Prof. E. Passarge, University of Essen School of Medicine, Essen, Germany.)

Hirschsprung disease is also the first multifactorial disorder for which the genetic causes have been well described (Table 9.1). *RET* (*re*arranged during *t*ransfection) (see Chapters 5 and 8) is one of 10 partially interdependent genes associated with HSCR. Mutations in both *RET* ligands—glial cell line–derived neurotrophic factor (*GDNF*) and neurturin (*NRTN*)—have been associated with HSCR, but primarily a mutation in *RET* also makes a multigenic contribution. Three other cellular pathways are also involved: the endothelin type B receptor (EDNRB) pathway, with its ligand endothelin-3 (EDN3) and endothelin-converting enzyme (ECE1); the SOX10 transcription pathway; and a MADH interacting protein. Five of the genes listed in Table 9.1 (*RET, EDNRB, EDN3, GDNF,* and *SOX10*) account for 60 to 70% of familial cases of HSCR and 10 to 30% of sporadic cases.

The phenotype associated with HSCR varies with the pathway. Diminished function of the RET pathway appears to result in isolated HSCR as a result of abnormal neural crest migration within the gut. Defects in the endothelin or SOX10 pathways result in HSCR and the melanocytic pigmentary defects found in Waardenburg syndrome (Fig. 9.5), which are consistent with a slightly broader impact on neural crest cell differentiation. Defects in the MADH interacting protein result in an even more upstream developmental effect with abnormal differentiation of cranial, vagal, and enteric neural crest cells through an as yet undefined mechanism. These mechanisms do not account for all cases of HSCR. It is likely that other contributions to these four pathways and various multigenic interactions will be discovered.

Neural Tube Defects

Neural tube defects (**NTDs**) are another set of multifactorial congenital disorders with a predicted recurrence risk of 3 to 4% in siblings. NTDs are caused by abnormal closure of the embryonic neural tube in week 3 or 4 of gestation (Fig. 9.6). The genetic contributions to normal closure are not fully described in humans, but more than 80 genes, contributing to everything from appropriate bending of the neural tube to closure of the neuropores, have been identified in mice. Specific environmental factors play a role in some cases. Investigators found that women who gave birth to children with NTDs had high homocysteine levels in their blood. As a result, folic acid supplementation was used empirically prior to conception and throughout the first 4 weeks of pregnancy, and it decreased the occurrence of NTDs by 50%.

Genes that may be involved in the etiology of neural tube defects include genes of folate and homocysteine metabolism (Box 9.1; Fig. 9.7). The methylenetetrahydrofolate reductase (*MTHFR*) gene has a 677C → T mutation that results in an ala22val substitution, and it is present in high frequencies in the population (30% of whites and 10% of African Americans). Individuals with spina bifida and their mothers are more likely to be homozygous for the mutation (sometimes designated as 677TT) than normal controls and their

TABLE 9.1 GENES IMPLICATED IN THE ETIOLOGY OF HIRSCHSPRUNG DISEASE

GENE	GENE PRODUCT AND FUNCTION	LOCATION	CONTRIBUTION TO HSCR	PENETRANCE
RET	Receptor tyrosine kinase Promotes neural crest stem cell migration in the intestines	10q11.2	Loss of function 50% of HSCR 75% with long segment disease	50–72%
GDNF	Glial cell line–derived neurotrophic factor RET ligand Role in neural crest stem cell migration?	5p13.1	Variants usually interact with *RET* variants to produce HSCR	Unknown
NRTN	Neurturin; *RET* ligand Promotes neuronal survival	19p13.3	Variants require interaction with *RET* variants to cause HSCR	Unknown
GFRA1	GDNF receptor alpha Binds GDNF and mediates activation of RET	10q26	Necessary for proper RET signaling No mutation identified yet	Unknown
EDNRB	Endothelin receptor type B	13q22	5% of HSCR 95% with short segment disease	30–85%
EDN3	Endothelin 3 Proliferation and melanogenesis in neural crest cells?	20q13.2–13.3	Heterozygote mutation: weak HSCR contribution Homozygote mutation: Waardenburg/HSCR	Unknown
ECE1	Endothelin-converting enzyme 1 Proteolytic processing of endothelin 3 to active peptide form	1p36.1	Heterozygote missense Skip lesions of HSCR	Unknown
SOX10	Acts in conjunction with PAX3 as transcriptional activator of *MITF* promoter; MITF controls development and postnatal survival of melanocytes	22q13	Dominant negative causes peripheral demyelinating neuropathy, central demyelinating leukodystrophy, Waardenburg syndrome, and HSCR	>80%
ZFHX1B	Zinc finger homeobox 1B; MADH-interacting protein 1 Needed for migration of cranial neural crest cells and development of vagal neural crest precursors (the precursors of the enteric nervous system)	2q22	<2% of HSCR Heterozygous null alleles cause Mowat-Wilson syndrome of seizures, agenesis of corpus callosum, congenital heart defects, and ± HSCR	Unknown

HSCR, Hirschsprung disease

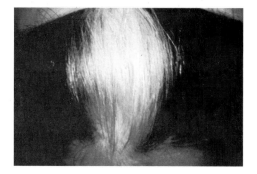

FIGURE 9.5 The white forelock frequently found in Waardenburg syndrome is a melanocytic pigmentary defect. Other characteristics of the syndrome include autosomal dominant inheritance, cochlear hearing loss, pigmentation abnormality of the iris, and early graying. Type 4, or Waardenburg-Shah syndrome, also has features of Hirschsprung disease and is associated with germline defects in the endothelin system or SOX10.

mothers. If both a mother and her child are homozygous and/or if the red blood cell folate level in the mother is in the lowest quartile, the odds ratio for having a child with an NTD is 3.28. Investigators reported that mothers who were homozygotes of a polymorphism of the methylenetetrahydrofolate dehydrogenase (*MTHFD*) gene (arg653gln) had a mildly increased risk of having a child with an NTD (odds ratio, 1.52). In the homocysteine–methionine cycle, polymorphisms in the genes for both methionine synthase and methionine synthase reductase influenced the risk of spina bifida if present in the mother, with the risk increasing in homozygotes as compared to heterozygotes. Cysteine β-synthase deficiency, an autosomal recessive disorder resulting in homocystinuria, has not been directly associated with an increased risk of NTDs; however, mouse embryos exposed to extremely high levels of homocysteine are relatively likely to develop NTDs. These findings are all described as associations, and the direct cause of NTDs has not yet been established.

In 1991, the U.S. Public Health Service recommended that all women who had given birth to a child with an NTD should take 4 mg/day of folic acid beginning 1 month before trying to become pregnant. In 1992, the U.S. Public Health Service modified this recommendation and urged that all women of childbearing age take 400 mcg of folic acid daily, because most pregnancies are unplanned. Once a woman is pregnant, the recommended daily allowance is 600 mcg, and during lactation, it is 500 mcg. In 1996, the Food and Drug Administration required that folic acid be added to most enriched breads, flours, corn meals, rice, noodles, pasta, and other grain products. The Centers for Disease Control and Prevention estimate that routine use of folic acid by all women of childbearing age would reduce the incidence of NTDs by as much as 70%. The incidence of NTDs in Canada decreased from 16.2 per 10,000 pregnancies before routine use of folic acid to 8.6 per 10,000 after routine use of folic acid was recommended.

ADULT-ONSET COMPLEX DISEASES

Cardiovascular Disease

The American Heart Association states that cardiovascular disease claims more lives annually than cancer, chronic lung disease, accidents, diabetes, and respiratory infections combined. Cardiovascular disease includes coronary artery disease (CAD), cardiomyopathies, conduction abnormalities, hypertension, stroke, aneurysm, and peripheral vascular disease, each of which has multiple genes of different natures that may contribute to disease incidence to varying degrees.

More than 50% of cases of cardiovascular disease are CAD. To date, most genes found to be involved in CAD have been identified using association studies. The same *MTHFR* gene allele (677C → T) that has been associated with an increased risk of NTDs is also associated with a 16% increased risk of premature CAD in homozygous persons and in conjunction with a low folate level.

The early genetic contributions to the pathogenesis of CAD and ultimately myocardial infarction are unknown except for a few contributing genes. In 2003, the first autosomal dominant form of CAD was described in one large extended family. The cause was a seven–amino acid deletion in transcription factor MEF2A (myocyte-specific enhancer factor 2), which normally binds to a DNA target sequence found in the regulator regions of most muscle-specific genes. The deletion disrupts the nuclear localization of MEF2A.

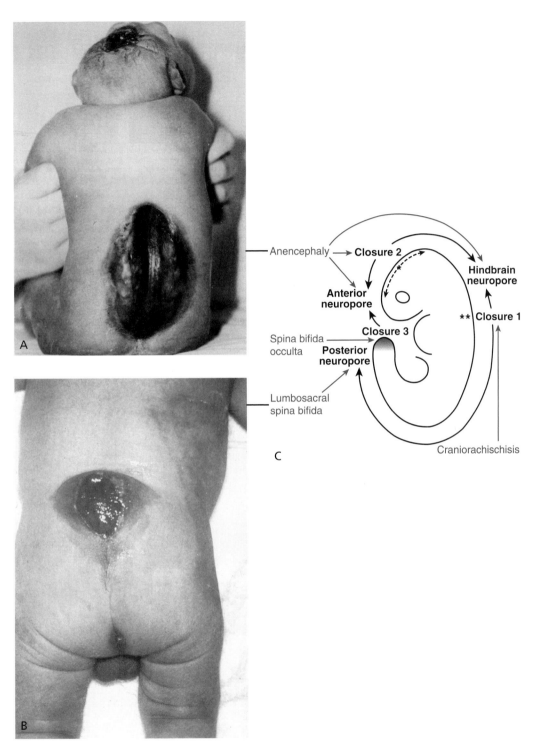

FIGURE 9.6 Neural tube defects caused by failure of closure of the embryonic neural tube at the anterior and posterior neuropores. **A.** Anencephaly and a severe rachischisis form of thoracolumbar spina bifida. **B.** Lumbosacral spina bifida. **C.** Neural tube closure sequence. Closure initiates at each of three regions (*closure 1, closure 2,* and *closure 3*) and then fuses intermittently in both directions toward the relative neuropores. A neural tube defect may result from failure either to initiate or to complete closure. (Part A reprinted with permission from Langman Medical Embryology, Baltimore: Williams & Wilkins, 1975. By permission from J. Warkany. Congenital Malformations. Year Book, Chicago, 1971. Part B reprinted with permission from Booth and Wezniak. Pediatrics, 1984. Distributed in the U.S. by Williams & Wilkins for Gower Medical Publishing. Image 209. Part C redrawn with permission from Copp AJ, Greene NDE, Murdoch JN. Nat Rev Genet 2003;4:784–793.)

BOX 9.1

Genes of Folate and Homocysteine Metabolism

- Genes of folate metabolism
  - Methylenetetrahydrofolate reductase (*MTHFR*)
  - Methylenetetrahydrofolate dehydrogenase (*MTHFD*)
- Genes of homocysteine metabolism
  - Methionine synthase (*MTR*)
  - Methionine synthase reductase (*MTRR*)
  - Cystathionine β-synthase (*CBS*)

Additional studies are necessary to determine whether *MEF2A* is an important contributor to CAD or only to a few families.

The genetics of highly penetrant cardiovascular diseases are just being explained, and the polygenic and allelic interactions will be described in the future. The study of cardiovascular genetics is approximately 10 years behind that of cancer genetics but will likely be the source of major genetic advances in the coming years.

Diabetes Mellitus

Type 1 diabetes mellitus is one of the most common chronic diseases of childhood, with a prevalence of 2 to 3 per 1000 in the 10- to 19-year age group. Selective autoimmune destruction of pancreatic islet β-cells results in lack of insulin production. A combination of genetic and undefined environmental influences such as viral infections has been implicated, and enteroviruses are most suspected. Pathogenesis is further affected by immune regulation and chemical mediators. At least 20 chromosomal regions have been linked to human susceptibility. The largest single contribution comes from several genes in the major histocompatibility complex at 6p21.3; this accounts for at least 40% of the familial aggregation of type 1 diabetes mellitus. Approximately 30% of patients with type 1 diabetes mellitus are heterozygous for HLA-DQ2/DQ8 (formerly known as HLA-DR3/DR4). In addition, HLA-DQ6 is associated with dominant protection from the disease.

Type 2 diabetes mellitus is the most common form of diabetes, affecting approximately 8% of adults in the United States. The body does not produce enough insulin, or insulin-resistance occurs at the target cell level. Type 2 diabetes mellitus is a heterogeneous disorder, similar to cancer, in that it is not a single disease

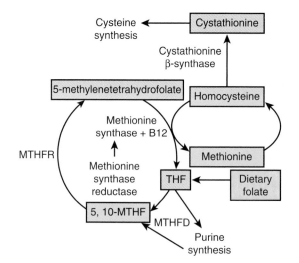

FIGURE 9.7 The folate–methionine metabolic pathway. MTHFR, methylenetetrahydrofolate reductase; MTHF, methylenetetrahydrofolate; THF, tetrahydrofolate; MTHFD, methylenetetrahydrofolate dehydrogenase. Vitamin B$_{12}$ (cobalamin) serves as a cofactor for methionine synthase.

but a group of metabolic disorders that have glucose intolerance in common. It is also considered a polygenic disorder with a complex interplay of factors that influence contributing traits such as β-cell mass, insulin secretion, insulin action, fat distribution, and obesity. Contributing environmental factors may influence the appearance of disease in genetically predisposed individuals. Some groups are at high risk, particularly African-American, American Indian, Asian-American, Pacific Island, and Hispanic-American populations. In 3234 people at high risk for type 2 diabetes mellitus, investigators found that moderate diet and exercise resulting in a 5 to 7% weight loss reduced the likelihood of disease by 60 to 70%. This study promoted lifestyle change as a significant prevention strategy.

Single-gene defects cause a minority of cases of type 2 diabetes mellitus. Glucokinase (*GCK* on 7p15-p13), which catalyzes the first step in glycolysis, is expressed only in liver and pancreatic islet β-cells. A loss-of-function mutation in one gene may produce symptoms of type 2 maturity-onset diabetes of the young (MODY). Type 2 MODY may present in children as mild hyperglycemia or in women as gestational diabetes and a family history of diabetes. The estimated prevalence of glucokinase deficiency in the United States is approximately 1 in 2500. About 50% of heterozygous women may develop gestational diabetes. Fewer than 50% of heterozygotes develop overt diabetes, and many of those are obese or elderly. Only 2% of patients with type 2 MODY require insulin therapy, and diabetes-associated complications are rare.

Types 1 and 3 MODY have similar clinical presentations but are associated with mutations in hepatocyte nuclear factor 4-α (*HNF4A* on 20q12-q13.1) and factor 1-α (*HNF1A* on 12q34). HNF4A, a member of the steroid hormone–thyroid hormone receptor superfamily, is expressed in liver, kidney, intestine, pancreatic islet cells, and insulinoma cells. It is an important regulator of hepatic gene expression and a major activator of HNF1A, which in turn activates the expression of a large number of liver-specific genes, such as those involved in glucose, cholesterol, and fatty acid metabolism.

Peroxisome proliferator–activated receptor-γ (*PPARγ* on 3p25) is a ligand-dependent transcription factor that regulates genes involved in lipid and glucose homeostasis along with adipocyte differentiation. The few individuals with a mutation in *PPARγ* have type 2 diabetes mellitus and excessive obesity. However, study of the transcription factor has improved our understanding of the association among type 2 diabetes mellitus, dyslipidemia, and atherosclerotic cardiovascular disease in diabetes in general. A new class of drugs, insulin-sensitizing thiazolidinediones, act as PPARγ agonists, decreasing the level of insulin resistance seen in many patients with type 2 diabetes mellitus. This may help prevent development of atherosclerotic plaques.

Alzheimer Disease

Alzheimer disease (AD) is the most common degenerative disorder of the central nervous system. It is estimated to affect 4 million people in the United States. The rate of AD occurrence is 2.8 per 1000 person-years in the 65- to 69-year age group, increasing to 56.1 per 1000 person-years in the over 90-year age group. In most affected individuals, dementia occurs after 65 years of age.

A small subgroup of people have AD associated with defects in one of three genes: amyloid precursor protein (*APP* on 21q21), presenilin 1 (*PSEN1* on 14q24.3), and presenilin 2 (*PSEN2* on 1q31-q42). More than 100 candidate genes have been evaluated, and only the e4 allele of the apolipoprotein E (*APOE*) gene has been consistently associated with increased susceptibility to develop AD.

APP is found in the cerebral cortical amyloid plaques in individuals with AD and in older individuals with Down syndrome. (*APP* is on 21q21 and is predicted to be synthesized in excess in individuals with trisomy 21.) As such, the gene was a logical candidate gene for familial AD. However, inherited mutations in *APP* have been found only in a small percentage of families with early-onset AD. Postmitotic mutations in neurons that result in dinucleotide deletions of microsatellite regions within *APP*, causing disruption of transcripts and abnormal protein aggregation, have been reported. With the lack of continuing mitosis, neurons may generate and accumulate abnormal proteins, leading to cellular disturbances and causing degeneration in sporadically occurring AD. This mechanism of postmitotic dinucleotide deletion at the transcript level may underlie a number of neurodegenerative pathologies. Presenilin 1 and presenilin 2 both appear to be γ-secretases functioning in different complexes but responsible for proteolytic cleavage of APP. Mutations in *PSEN1* are found in 18 to 50% of cases of autosomal dominant early-onset AD.

Apolipoprotein E (APOE), a main apoprotein of the chylomicron, binds to a specific receptor on liver cells and peripheral cells. APOE has been divided into three subtypes (e2, e3, and e4) based on electrophoretic properties. The most common apolipoprotein is *APOE e3*, which has been designated the wild-type genetic sequence. *APOE e4* differs from *APOE e3* at one position (cys112 → arg). *APOE e2* may differ from *APOE e3* at one of four locations. Homozygosity for *APOE e2* (e2e2) results in a low-penetrance risk of

familial dysbetalipoproteinemia or type III hyperlipoproteinemia (1–4%). The *APOE e4* allele is associated with the late-onset familial and sporadic forms of AD. The relative risk of AD associated with *APOE e4* homozygosity is increased in all ethnic groups compared to *APOE e3* homozygosity (African American, 3.0; white, 7.3; and Hispanic, 2.5). The risk is also increased for *APOE e4* heterozygosity in whites and Hispanics, but not necessarily in African Americans. In African Americans with AD, each copy of the e4 allele was associated with a 3.6-year earlier onset of disease. The results fit a clear linear dose–response relationship, with mean age of onset being 77.9 years with no e4 alleles, 74.3 years with 1 allele, and 70.7 years with 2 alleles.

In addition, *APOE e4* may modify the effects of the highly penetrant AD genes. One large Colombian family with a *PSEN1* mutation demonstrated that family members with at least one *APOE e4* allele were more likely to develop AD at an earlier age than those without an *APOE e4* allele.

ETHICS	Genetic Testing of Children Who Are at Risk for Adult-Onset Disorders

Genetic tests may be categorized by considering the clinical validity of the test and the availability of effective treatment for individuals who test positive. If the test has high clinical validity and effective treatment is available, such as for the multiple endocrine neoplasia type 2 syndromes (MEN2A, MEN2B, familial medullary thyroid carcinoma), familial adenomatous polyposis (FAP), or phenylketonuria (PKU), the concern is that testing be made available for eligible individuals to promote the best medical care. If a test has limited clinical validity but treatment is very effective, (e.g., *HFE* mutation testing for hereditary hemochromatosis), it may identify a person who is susceptible to the disease in question but will never actually develop it. However, appropriate screening can be initiated so that treatment is begun prior to the onset of irreversible complications. If a test has a high clinical validity for a disease with no treatment options (e.g., presymptomatic testing for Huntington disease), medical practitioners should be most concerned that adequate nondirective counseling is provided to allow at-risk persons to make an informed, autonomous decision. A test may have both limited clinical validity and no available effective treatment (e.g., *APOE e4* testing for AD).

Tests for MEN2, FAP, and PKU also have implications for children, because treatment should be initiated in childhood or infancy. Therefore, practitioners typically have no hesitation in obtaining the tests on minors. What about disorders that do not manifest themselves until adulthood?

ETHICS	Genetic Testing of Children Who Are at Risk for Adult-Onset Disorders *(continued)*

Suppose a woman comes for counseling with her 10-year-old son Nathan. She says she would like Nathan to be tested for Alzheimer disease and the *APOE e4* allele because "his father has Alzheimer disease in the early stages, we're divorcing, and if Nathan has it, I want to make sure his father doesn't get any visitation rights" (see Chapter 5).

When the practitioner is faced with a request to perform genetic testing for an adult-onset disorder in a child, several questions should be addressed:

- Will the child be the primary beneficiary of the test results?
- Is the child, not the parent, capable of understanding the implications of the result?
- Will the child be harmed physically or psychosocially if a gene mutation is identified?

In this situation, Nathan's mother is the primary beneficiary of the results because she would use them in a custody battle. Nathan might be kept from seeing and interacting with his father. From the information given, it cannot be determined whether that would be beneficial or detrimental. Most 10-year-old boys are not capable of the abstract long-range thinking necessary to understand the long-term implications of a diagnosis of Alzheimer disease. If Nathan is homozygous for the *APOE e4* allele, will his guardian mother treat him the same as she has in the past, or will she convey to Nathan some of her hostility toward Nathan's father? Will she expose Nathan to either negative or positive compensatory behavior because of the test result? Will Nathan face employment and insurance discrimination while the AD is in the presymptomatic stages?

Parents do not have a constitutionally protected right to demand that a practitioner perform a genetic test if the practitioner is unwilling. There is little risk of liability unless the child suffers physical harm as a result of the physician's refusal to perform the test.

Testing a child for Alzheimer disease may be highly theoretical, because most genetic professionals do not recommend it even for adults. However, we must always be aware of the slippery slope. If you would not test a child for Alzheimer disease, would you test him or her for Huntington disease? (Nathan's case was actually derived from a request for Huntington disease testing.) Should you test a young girl for hereditary breast/ovarian cancer syndrome, even though she is not likely to have risk for cancer until she is in her 20s?

USMLE-Style Questions

1. Newborn twins, both males, are delivered. One child is entirely normal. The other has a cleft lip and palate but has no other anomalies and appears developmentally appropriate. Neither parent has a cleft lip or palate. Both parents have normal intelligence and physical appearance. A karyotype of the affected child shows 46,XY. Study of DNA tandem repeats shows an identical fragment pattern between the two newborns. Which of the following is the appropriate explanation of this birth defect?

   a. Autosomal recessive syndrome in dizygotic twins
   b. Complex disorder with differential uterine environmental exposure
   c. De novo autosomal dominant germline mutation in the mother
   d. Questionable paternity
   e. X-linked recessive syndrome in dizygotic twins

Questions 2 and 3. This table shows con-cordance rates for three disorders in monozygotic twins, dizygotic twins, and siblings.

DISORDER	CONCORDANCE		
	MONOZYGOTIC TWINS (%)	DIZYGOTIC TWINS (%)	SIBLINGS (%)
A	100	25	25.0
B	50	6	6.0
C	10	10	0.1

2. Which one of the following causative patterns describes disorder C?
   a. Almost purely genetic, probably autosomal dominant
   b. Almost purely genetic, probably autosomal recessive
   c. Multifactorial with a strong genetic component
   d. Primarily environmental, with a postnatal environmental role
   e. Primarily environmental, with a prenatal environmental role

3. Which one of the following causative patterns describes disorder A?
   a. Almost purely genetic, probably autosomal dominant
   b. Almost purely genetic, probably autosomal recessive
   c. Multifactorial with a strong genetic component
   d. Primarily environmental, with a postnatal environmental role
   e. Primarily environmental, with a prenatal environmental role

Questions 4 and 5. This table summarizes risks that an individual will be affected with a disease according to its presence in a particular relative or population group.

DISEASE	IDENTICAL TWINS (%)	FIRST-DEGREE RELATIVES (%)	SECOND-DEGREE RELATIVES (%)	THIRD-DEGREE RELATIVES (%)	GENERAL POPU-LATION (%)
Cleft lip, palate	38–40	3.0–4.0	0.7–0.8	0.30	0.10
Club foot	30–32	2.5	0.5	0.20	0.10
Congenital hip dis-location	33	5.0	0.6	0.40	0.20
Type 1 diabetes mellitus	50	50	—	—	0.50
Type 2 diabetes mellitus	—	10.0–15.0	—	—	2.0–5.0
Schizophrenia	44–79	5.0–10.0	2.7	—	0.5
Autism	92	4.5	0.1	0.05	0.04

4. A father with cleft lip and palate has two normal children. According to the table, the risk that his next child will have a cleft lip and palate is
   a. 0.1%
   b. 3–4%
   c. 4–6%
   d. 5–10%
   e. 38–40%

5. An adopted man discovers a biological relative and obtains his family history. He discovers that he had an identical twin who was diagnosed with schizophrenia and that another of their five biological

siblings also had schizophrenia. According to the table, his risk of developing schizophrenia is approximately

- a. 0.5%
- b. 2.7%
- c. 5–10%
- d. 44%
- e. More than 44%

SUGGESTED READINGS

Clayton D, McKeigue PM. Epidemiological methods for studying genes and environmental factors in complex diseases. Lancet 2001;358:1356–1360.

Box NF, Duffy DL, Chen W, et al. MC1R genotype modifies risk of melanoma in families segregating CDKN2A mutations. Am J Hum Genet 2001;69:765–773.

Hall JG. Twinning. Lancet 2003;362:735–743.

Fairfield KM, Fletcher RH. Vitamins for chronic disease prevention in adults: scientific review. JAMA 2002;287:3116–3126.

Klerk M, Verhoef P, Clarke R, et al. MTHFR 677C → T polymorphism and risk of coronary heart disease: a meta-analysis. JAMA 2002;288:2023–2031.

Sturm AS. Cardiovascular genetics: are we there yet? J Med Genet 2004;41:321–323.

Bloch M, Hayden MR. Opinion: predictive testing for Huntington disease in childhood: challenges and implications. Am J Hum Genet 1990;46:1–4.

Harper PS, Clarke A. Should we test children for "adult" genetic diseases? Lancet 1990;335:1205–1206.

WEB RESOURCES

http://www.cdc.gov/node.do/id/0900f3ec80010af9
Department of Health and Human Resources, Centers for Disease Control and Prevention. Fact sheets on folic acid usage. Includes a link to "Babies and Birth Defects: A Mystery in Texas," an educational module designed to teach middle school and high school students about epidemiology, neural tube birth defects, and folic acid.

http://diabetes.niddk.nih.gov/index.htm
National Diabetes Information Clearinghouse, National Institute of Diabetes and Digestive and Kidney Diseases (NIDDK) of the National Institutes of Health.

http://nihseniorhealth.gov/listoftopics.html
National Institute on Aging, National Institutes of Health. Resource for information on Alzheimer disease.

Developmental Genetics

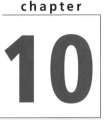
DYSMORPHOLOGY
EMBRYOLOGICAL DEVELOPMENT AND
   CONTROL MECHANISMS
     Early Development
     Transcription Factors
       HOX *Genes*
       TBX *Genes*
       GATA *Genes*

Induction and Morphogens
Sex Differentiation and Intersex
   Conditions
USMLE-STYLE QUESTIONS

The study of meiosis and then cytogenetics led initially to the investigation of the earliest stages of human development, and the study of embryology has historically been an observational field dealing with the progression in structure of the developing human embryo. This observational methodology continued into the fetal, neonatal, and childhood periods with **dysmorphology,** the study of morphological developmental abnormalities seen in many syndromes of genetic, multifactorial, or environmental origin. The molecular basis of normal embryological development and mutations with subsequent dysmorphology is difficult to discover in humans but has the potential to expand our knowledge of the complexities of the human genome and its control mechanisms.

DYSMORPHOLOGY

Dysmorphology does not seek to define what is normal but to discover what is most common and what differs in ways that result in abnormal function. In many cases, conventions developed by portrait artists have been used. Physical measurements of body parts have been obtained, and statistical comparisons have been made within the general population, between males and females, within age groups, and within various ethnic groups. Data concerning the size, proportion, and relative posi-

tioning of all facial features as well as extremities and upper body to lower body relationships are available. Individuals are considered "dysmorphic" only if their proportions or measurements are more than two standard deviations from the norm. (Traditionally, it was common among some practitioners to refer to the dysmorphic child as an "FLK" or "funny-looking kid" and even to include such terminology in the medical record. Put yourself in the place of a parent of a dysmorphic child and consider the lack of professionalism displayed by using a pejorative term to refer to such a patient.)

Dysmorphology in a fetus, neonate, or child provides clues to the embryological development of the individual. A major malformation or "birth defect"—one requiring significant surgical or medical intervention—is obvious (Box 10.1). Every individual has one or two minor dysmorphic features or minor malformations. When three or more minor malformations occur in the same individual, it may be a sign of an underlying genetic or multifactorial condition that may benefit from intervention. Dysmorphic features in an older child or an adult are more difficult to interpret because environmental effects may be superimposed onto developmental changes.

The evaluation of an individual for dysmorphic features involves a systematic approach to

---

BOX 10.1

Types of Major Birth Defects

- **Malformation:** structural defect resulting from an intrinsically abnormal developmental process
- **Disruption:** structural defect resulting from the breakdown of or interference with an originally normal developmental process
- **Deformation:** abnormality in form or position of a body part caused by a nondisruptive mechanical force (mechanical constraint or secondary effects from another abnormality in the fetus)
- **Dysplasia:** abnormal organization of cells into tissues and its morphological consequence
- **Sequence:** structural defect or mechanical factor that leads to multiple secondary effects
- **Syndrome:** multiple anomalies with a single basic cause that occur independently rather than sequentially

---

the entire physical examination, with extra attention paid to the head, ears, eyes, nose and throat, hands and feet, body proportions, and genitalia. The remainder of the examination is very similar to a routine medical evaluation. It is essential that all appropriate examination findings be recorded. Physical measurements should be taken and recorded. Features should be described in writing, even if they are apparently normal. Written descriptions stating that a feature is "normal" or "WNL" for "within normal limits" should be used cautiously. (Use of "WNL" may be interpreted in some circles as "we never looked.") A well-written evaluation should not require accompanying photographic corroboration. Table 10.1 includes written descriptions of normal and dysmorphic features. The language of dysmorphology may require that the student refer to a medical dictionary.

Dysmorphology may also be referred to as syndromology, because the observed phenotypes have been described and given eponymous syndrome designations prior to determination of a molecular or environmental cause. If a syndrome has been named after an affected individual, the appropriate designation is "Name's syndrome" (possessive form). If a syndrome has been named after the unaffected reporter, the designation is "Name syndrome" (no possessive). As the underlying causes for syndromes have been discovered, some eponyms are no longer commonly used. For example, Edwards syndrome has become known as trisomy 18, but Down syndrome has maintained equal footing with the causative designation trisomy 21. Other conditions change names as our knowledge of pathogenesis improves. Potter syndrome occurs in a fetus with bilateral renal agenesis, resulting in markedly decreased or absent amniotic fluid and secondary pulmonary hypoplasia and skeletal deformations. This disorder is now more properly referred to as Potter sequence.

With the advent of molecular genetics, many entities that were once identified by dysmorphologists and other physicians as separate diseases and syndromes have been determined to be caused by defects in the same gene (e.g., achondroplasia, thanatophoric dysplasia, and hypochondroplasia; multiple endocrine neoplasia type 2 and Hirschsprung disease). Dysmorphology has opened doors of understanding of human development, permitting a systematic description of physical phenotypes.

EMBRYOLOGICAL DEVELOPMENT AND CONTROL MECHANISMS

Evaluation of dysmorphic features requires understanding of embryological principles and patterns, and understanding of the molecular cause requires knowledge of the developmental genetics behind the embryological observations. Much research is yet to be done in human developmental genetics.

Early Development

The fertilized egg, or zygote, and the first 2 to 4 cells in the embryo are **totipotent,** meaning

TABLE 10.1 USE OF DESCRIPTIVE LANGUAGE FOR EVALUATION OF DYSMORPHIC FEATURES BASED ON ARTISTS' NORMS

EXAMINATION AREA	NORMAL NEWBORN	NEWBORN WITH DOWN SYNDROME
Head	Prominent occiput with slightly overriding cranial sutures. Anterior fontanel flat, patent, and 2 × 2 cm. Posterior fontanel open and fingertip sized.	Mild brachycephaly. Anterior fontanel flat, patent and 2 × 2 cm. Posterior fontanel open and fingertip sized.
Eyes	Normal palpebral fissures, globes, and spacing. No epicanthal folds. Red reflex ×2.	Up-slanting palpebral fissures, bilateral epicanthal folds. Normal interpupillary distance. Red reflex ×2.
Ears	Normal size and position. Tympanic membranes obscured by vernix.	Ears somewhat small, with folded superior margins of helices. Tympanic membranes obscured by vernix.
Nose	Normal nose and nasal bridge. Both nares patent.	Flat nasal bridge with small nasal bones. Both nares patent.
Throat	Normal tongue structure and mobility, good suck reflex (typically part of neuro section)	Protruding tongue, normal size. Decreased suck reflex.
Genitalia	Normal female external genitalia. Labia separated.	Normal male genitalia. No hypospadias or chordae. Both testes descended.
Extremities	Digits normal. Single transverse palmar crease on right hand. Good movement of all 4 extremities. No evidence of hip clicks or congenital hip dysplasia.	Bilateral 5th finger clinodactyly, bilateral single transverse palmar creases. Broad space between 1st and 2nd toes. Hips preferentially in abducted position. No evidence of hip clicks or congenital hip dysplasia.

Additional detail may be added by including actual physical measurements.

that they have the potential to develop into a complete organism. The zygote does not transcribe mRNA initially until the 4- to 8-cell stage. A variety of maternal mRNAs stored in oocytes in an inactive form and activated after fertilization provide the initial translation activities of the cells. It is not known whether there is an association between loss of totipotency and initiation of transcription, but around this time, cells begin the process of cellular determination in which stable changes occur that determine the lineage. Certainly, determination has occurred at or before random X-inactivation in the female embryo.

Differentiation follows, and cell types are formed with structural and functional specialization at about the 16-cell stage, resulting in cells that are destined for either the embryo and amnion (inner cell mass) or for the chorion and the embryo's contribution to the placenta (trophoblast). It is not known exactly how the differentiation is initiated, but the relative position of a cell within the cluster of cells and the relative impact of direct cell-to-cell signaling may be involved. Cells of the inner cell mass can give rise to all of the cells of the embryo but can no longer produce the trophoblast, meaning that they are **pluripo-**

tent. Formation of identical twins is due to division of the totipotent embryo or the pluripotent inner cell mass. The paternal and maternal genomes have their own parent-of-origin methylation in their imprinted genes that are reset through genome-wide demethylation in the preimplantation embryo.

The cells of the inner cell mass give rise to the germ layers of ectoderm, mesoderm, and endoderm. Once differentiation is under way, gene expression in the various cell lines is preserved through epigenetic modifications in a semipermanent manner, providing a form of cell memory in succeeding cell divisions. De novo methylation occurs prior to the differentiation of ectoderm, mesoderm, and endoderm. Lineages that give rise to the trophoblast remain undermethylated; somatic cell lineages are heavily methylated; and early primordial germ cells remain unmethylated until after the gonads differentiate.

None of the germ layer cells is able to produce an entire embryo, but each is **multipotent,** having the ability to give rise to a specific range of cell types. Cells in different germ layers cannot produce cell types produced by another layer. Eventually, **unipotent** cells arise; they can produce only a single type of differentiated cell. A precursor cell that is capable of self-renewal as a continual source of differentiated cells is a **stem cell.** Stem cells are classified in terms of their potency: totipotent; pluripotent, or embryonic; multipotent; or unipotent.

Although differentiation results in specific cell types, **morphogenesis** is the process whereby the shape of the embryo is generated. The embryo must also develop with an axis (craniocaudal, anteroposterior) and laterality (right–left). The determinant of this asymmetry is uncertain in humans but may involve the site of sperm entry into the ovum. In addition to epigenetic factors, differentiation results from differential gene expression that is controlled, at least in part, by transcription factors. (Except in lymphocytes, differential gene expression is not a result of loss of DNA within the cell.) Clusters of families of transcription factors contribute to the development of the asymmetry of the embryo.

Transcription Factors

HOX Genes

One family of developmental transcription factors, **HOX genes,** or *homeotic box* genes, is named for their similarity to *Drosophila* genes that are responsible for the appropriate segmentation of the insect's body. When these genes mutate, one body part develops with the appearance of another (legs where the antennae should be). These segmental genes code for proteins that contain a structural motif of three linked α-helices (or homeodomain) in the helix-turn-helix family of DNA-binding proteins. Humans have 39 *HOX* genes in four clusters on four chromosomes in a temporospatial arrangement (Fig. 10.1). Each gene has two exons, the second of which contains the 180-bp homeodomain coding region, or homeo box. The gene cluster regions have the lowest frequency of repeat fragments in the genome, effectively preserving the coding and control sequences.

Two *HOX* genes, *HOXD13* and *HOXA13*, are mutated in human malformation syndromes and participate in the development of the most caudal structures of the body—the hands, feet, and genital tubercle. The phenotypes are subtle. With *HOXD13* mutations, there is syndactyly of the third and fourth fingers and an extra digit (polydactyly). With *HOXA13* mutations, there may be hypoplastic thumbs, short fingers, urinary tract malformations, male hypospadias, or defective female müllerian duct fusion. Subtle changes in phenotype are seen if the mutation is a simple loss-of-function mutation or a dominant negative mutation. Somatic mutations of *HOXA9* have been associated with the development of leukemia. *HOX* genes may be overexpressed in solid tumors that originate from tissues in which the *HOX* genes are normally expressed.

TBX Genes

Another family of phylogenetically conserved transcription factors are the T-box genes (*TBX*). *TBX* genes play roles in the differentiation of the three germ layers and in later organogenesis, with particular expression in cardiac and pharyngeal arch development.

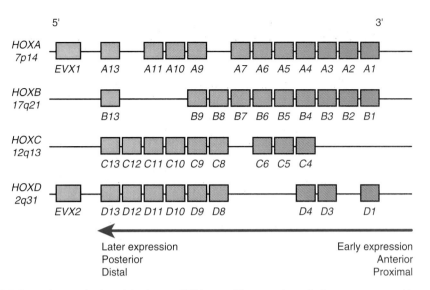

FIGURE 10.1 Genomic organization of the human *HOX* genes. The genes in each cluster are arranged in order from both a temporal and spatial perspective. Genes at the 3′ end are expressed early in cranial and proximal regions. Genes at the 5′ end are expressed later in more caudal and distal regions. (Adapted with permission from Goodman FR. Limb malformations and the human HOX genes. Am J Med Genet 2002;112:256–265.)

Three separate clinical phenotypes have been localized to chromosome 22q11.2; they are referred to as del22q11.2 (Box 10.2). Molecular studies have shown that del22q11.2 is relatively frequent, occurring in 1 in 4000 live births, with a highly variable dominant phenotype even within families. The *TBX1* gene is in the middle of the 22q11.2 critical region. Mutations resulting in haploinsufficiency of *TBX1* have been found in individuals with features of the del22q11.2 syndrome but without the 1.5- to 3-Mb deletion found in 96% of affected individuals.

In mice, *Tbx1* is found in the pharyngeal endoderm in a craniocaudal wave of expression. *Tbx1* expression is thought to initiate the invagination of endodermal cells toward the ectoderm, forming the pharyngeal pouches. If *Tbx1* is not expressed, the endoderm remains straight, and no pouch forms. The pharyngeal endoderm of the pouches contributes to the parathyroids and thymus. The pharyngeal pouch arteries run inside the pharyngeal arches, and the third, fourth, and sixth pharyngeal arch arteries combine to form the mature aortic arch. *Tbx1* has been found to have an additional role in supporting the

growth of the fourth pharyngeal arch artery. The more cranial pharyngeal arches themselves contribute to head and neck structures (first arch, maxilla and mandible; second arch, hyoid bone). Virtually all of these structures of the pharyngeal arches, pouches, and arteries may be affected in the del22q11.2 phenotype.

Holt-Oram syndrome is a dominant disorder characterized by a defect in cardiac septation, usually an atrial septal defect, and a thumb anomaly, either absence of the digit or a triphalangeal, nonopposable, fingerlike digit (Fig. 10.2). The upper extremity abnormality may be as mild as fusion of the carpal bones or as severe as phocomelia with the hand attached close to the trunk. An individual with Holt-Oram syndrome and a translocation involving 12q2 provided the approximate location of the gene, which has been identified as *TBX5* at 12q24.1. TBX5 interacts synergistically with the transcription factor product of a cardiac-specific homeobox gene (*NKX2.5*) to promote cardiomyocyte differentiation. Loss-of-function mutations result in haploinsufficiency, with some genotype–phenotype correlation. Null alleles produce

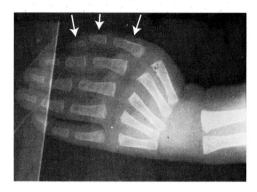

FIGURE 10.2 Triphalangeal thumb seen in Holt-Oram syndrome. Three ossification centers are present in the thumb (*arrows*). (Reprinted with permission from Famous Teachings in Modern Medicine, Syndromes in Pediatrics Part II, 1971, with permission from Medcom, Inc.)

> **BOX 10.2**
>
> ## 22q11.2 deletion syndromes
>
> - CATCH22
>   - Cardiac Abnormality, abnormal facies
>   - T cell deficit due to thymic hypoplasia
>   - Cleft palate
>   - Hypocalcemia due to hypoparathyroidism
> - DiGeorge syndrome (pharyngeal pouch III and IV syndrome)
>   - Parathyroid hypoplasia with neonatal hypocalcemia
>   - Thymic hypoplasia
>   - Cardiac outflow tract defects (tetralogy of Fallot, truncus arteriosus, interrupted aortic arch, right aortic arch, aberrant right subclavian artery)
> - Velocardial facial syndrome (Shprintzen syndrome)
>   - Cleft palate (overt or submucous)
>   - Cardiac anomalies
>   - Typical facies
>   - Learning disabilities
> - Conotruncal anomaly face syndrome
>   - Cardiac outflow tract defects (tetralogy of Fallot, pulmonary atresia, double-outlet right ventricle, truncus arteriosus communis, and aortic arch anomalies)
>   - Typical facies

severe cardiac and skeletal defects. Mutations at the C-terminal end of the T-box cause mild cardiac defects but severe skeletal anomalies. Missense mutations at the amino terminus of the T-box DNA-binding domain cause severe cardiac defects but milder skeletal anomalies, probably through inability to interact with NKX2.5. By itself, NKX2.5 is important for regulation of septation during cardiac morphogenesis and for maturation and maintenance of atrioventricular node function throughout life.

GATA Genes

A member of another group of transcription factors, the GATA-binding proteins, also interacts in cardiac differentiation. The members of this family recognize a GATA consensus sequence found in the promoters of many genes and contain one or two zinc-finger motifs for DNA binding.

- *GATA1* regulates expression of genes critical for erythroid development, such as the globin genes.
- *GATA2* has been implicated in the regulation of endothelial gene expression and hematopoiesis.
- *GATA3* appears to control expression of T-cell receptor genes.
- *GATA4* is expressed in yolk sac endoderm and cells involved in heart formation during fetal development.

A heterozygous missense mutation of *GATA4* has been found in a large family with isolated cardiac septal defects. DNA-binding affinity and transcriptional activity were reduced, and a physical interaction between GATA4 and TBX5 was eliminated. The interaction of T-box genes, cardiac-specific homeobox genes, and the GATA-binding proteins illustrate the complexities of developmental genetics and embryonic patterning.

Induction and Morphogens

Transcription factors must be activated in some fashion. For instance, the initial transcription and expression of homeodomain proteins is coordinated through a response to retinoic acid, a common inductive signal in embryonic development. Small hydrophobic hormones and morphogens, such as steroid hormones, thyroxine, and retinoic acid, diffuse through the plasma membranes and bind to intracellular receptors that are inducible transcription factors.

Retinoic acid also functions as a **morphogen** whose release at a position in the embryo creates a concentration gradient, with high concentrations of morphogen close to the source and low concentrations away from the source. The process by which one part of an embryo causes adjacent tissues to change through diffusion of substances is **induction.** The morphogen gradient leads to different cell fates. Morphogens may also be released in a series of signals provided by different agents (**sequential induction**).

The classic example of a morphogen gradient is the development of the vertebrate limb bud. Specific human data are lacking but have been inferred because of the degree of genetic homology in chicks, mice, and humans. Limb development includes such diverse processes as three-dimensional patterning (proximodistal, anteroposterior, and dorsoventral), cartilage and bone differentiation, and programmed cell death. It is regulated by a complex network of signal molecules that work in concert. The anteroposterior distribution of the type of digits involves the signaling protein **sonic hedgehog** (*SHH* on 7q36) emanating from the zone of polarizing activity at the posterior margin of the limb (Fig. 10.3). In addition, *SHH* is 1expressed in the Hensen node, the floor plate of the neural tube, the early gut endoderm, and throughout the notochord. *SHH* has also been implicated as the key inductive signal in patterning of the ventral neural tube and the ventral somites. The mechanism of action of *SHH* in the limb bud is not completely understood, but it appears to require a local asymmetrical expression pattern. If another center of expression occurs, polydactyly develops.

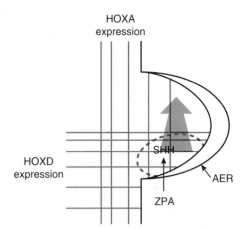

FIGURE 10.3 Limb bud induction mechanisms. *HOXA* and *HOXD* genes are expressed in the limb buds. Five *HOXA* genes are expressed in a proximodistal pattern and five *HOXD* genes, in an anteroposterior pattern. SHH released from the zone of polarizing activity (ZPA) at the posterior margin forms a morphogen gradient. SHH induces a feedback loop with the apical ectodermal ridge (AER), the primary source of fibroblast growth factor 4 (FGF4).

SHH is expressed in the midline of the embryo in the mesoderm, shortly after the three germ layers are formed. It is required for both the induction of the floor plate of the axial neural tube and the differentiation of a portion of the forebrain (rostral diencephalon). A second compound, a member of the transforming growth factor-β (TGF-β) family (BMP7, bone morphogenetic protein 7), is present in the midline mesoderm of the forebrain as well, and both SHH and BMP7 are necessary for proper forebrain differentiation. An SHH gradient is present from the mesoderm through the neuroectoderm and ectoderm and directs the patterning of the neural tube. A sequential induction may also exist, wherein SHH induces additional signals that perpetuate the signal. SHH has several actions during central nervous system development, including the differentiation of oligodendrocytes, proliferation of neural precursors, and control of axon growth.

Heterozygous mutations in *SHH* have been found to cause holoprosencephaly, the most common developmental defect of the forebrain and midface, with a frequency of 1 in 16,000 live births. Holoprosencephaly may show variable expressivity, from the extremely mild facial phenotype of a single central maxillary incisor and mild hypotelorism to classical holoprosencephaly (Fig. 10.4), and to cyclopia (single eye with a proboscis on the forehead above the eye). Genetic heterogeneity exists. Holoprosencephaly may be seen in trisomy 13 and also in mutations of the *ZIC2* gene (zinc-finger protein of cerebellum 2) found on 13q32. ZIC2 is expressed on the ectodermal surface side of the developing forebrain more distant from the developing midface; associated facial anomalies are rare with *ZIC2* mutations. *SIX3* (sine oculus

homeobox) on 2p21, which is expressed in the anterior portion of the developing neural tube, is necessary for proper forebrain and eye development and is mutated in some individuals with holoprosencephaly. Two additional genes have less penetrance and may serve as modifier genes: *TGIF* (TGF-β–induced factor) and *DKK1* ("Dickkopf," or big head).

Mutations in different components of a single signaling pathway may result in the same clinical condition. The transmembrane protein PTCH ("patched," on 9q22.3) normally inhibits transcription of the *TGF-β* and *Wnt* gene families through a signaling cascade. When SHH binds to PTCH, the inhibition is lifted and transcription occurs. If a mutation occurs in *PTCH*, SHH may not be able to bind effectively or the signaling cascade may be disrupted, effectively generating an SHH-deficient phenotype. In fact, mutations in *PTCH* have been shown to produce holoprosencephaly. If PTCH inhibition is not released, apoptosis of neuroectodermal cells occurs.

Sex Differentiation and Intersex Conditions

Sex determination results from the genetic sex of the embryo (46,XY or 46,XX) and its interaction with the developing gonads, internal genital ducts, and external genital structures. The genetic sex determines whether the primordial gonad differentiates into a testis or ovary. Differentiation is extremely complex. The exact order of differentiation has not been completely elucidated, but certain components have been determined through the study of individuals with intersex conditions. (The term *intersex condition* is used in this text. The terms hermaphroditism and male or female pseudohermaphroditism are historical, do not accurately describe the pathophysiology, and are frequently misinterpreted and misunderstood by practitioners and patients.)

A single Y-related gene, *SRY* (sex-determining region Y), acts as a switch signal for testis differentiation. It is unusual among human genes in that it is 3.8 kb long and has no introns. *SRY* encodes a transcription factor that is a member of the high-mobility group (HMG)

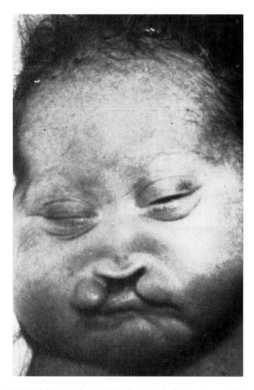

FIGURE 10.4 Infant with classical holoprosencephaly. Notice decreased distance between the palpebral fissures (hypotelorism), extremely flat nose with likely absence of nasal bones, and midline cleft lip and palate. According to artists' standards, the distance between the palpebral fissures should be approximately the length of one palpebral fissure. The underlying brain abnormality is a single midline cerebral ventricle with lack of development of the midline cerebral structures. Death usually occurs in the neonatal period. (Reprinted from *Famous Teachings in Modern Medicine, Syndromes in Pediatrics Part I*, 1972, with permission from Medcom, Inc.)

box family of DNA-binding proteins. The HMG-box binds to specific target sequences in DNA and is able to bend and unwind the chromatin. DNA bending appears to be part of the mechanism through which *SRY* influences transcription of other genes and initiates a cascade of gene interactions, ultimately leading to the formation of a testis from the indifferent fetal gonad.

Testis development is also controlled by genes on chromosomes other than the Y. For instance, the product of *WT1* (Wilms tumor gene 1) on 11p13 activates *SRY* by binding to its promoter region. *WT1* encodes a zinc-finger DNA-binding protein that is required for normal formation of the genitourinary system and mesothelial tissues. Alternative splicing, RNA editing, and the use of alternative translation initiation sites generate more than 30 isoforms of *WT1*. Individuals with dominant negative germline mutations in zinc-finger 3 or 4 of *WT1* may have Denys-Drash syndrome, consisting of Wilms tumor, nephropathy, and XX or XY gonadal dysgenesis. WT1 isoforms associate and synergize with steroidogenic factor-1 (SF-1), a nuclear receptor that regulates the transcription of a number of genes involved in reproduction, steroidogenesis, and male sexual differentiation. The interaction of WT1 and SF-1 promotes antimüllerian hormone expression from the Sertoli cells, resulting in regression of the müllerian ducts, which would otherwise differentiate into the uterus and fallopian tubes. Mutations in the genes for the antimüllerian hormone or the antimüllerian hormone receptor may cause persistent müllerian duct syndrome in otherwise normal males. The typical presentation is undescended testes, bilateral inguinal hernias, and normal external male genitalia. A uterus and fallopian tubes are present along with testes.

One of the earliest effects of SRY expression is to induce upregulation in the developing gonad of an autosomal gene, the SRY-related HMG-box gene *SOX9* on 17q24.3–25.1. Before sexual differentiation, SOX9 protein is found in the cytoplasm of undifferentiated gonads from both sexes. At the time of testis differentiation and antimüllerian hormone

expression, it becomes localized to the nuclear compartment in the genital ridges in males, whereas it is downregulated in females. *SOX9* is also expressed during chondrocyte differentiation and interacts with the collagen gene *COL2A1*. Infants with haploinsufficiency due to a heterozygous loss-of-function mutation in *SOX9* have camptomelic dysplasia, a disorder characterized by congenital bowing (*campto*) of long bones with a female phenotype in XY infants.

Luteinizing hormone stimulates formation of Leydig cells and secretion of testosterone. Homozygous loss-of-function mutations in the luteinizing hormone/choriogonadotropin receptor gene (*LHCGR* on 2p21) produce phenotypes that correlate to the amount of function lost. The severe form is associated with female external genitalia, absent müllerian structures, and undescended testes in XY individuals. XX individuals have primary amenorrhea or oligomenorrhea, cystic ovaries, and infertility.

Development of the female phenotype cannot be considered a default process. The nuclear hormone receptor gene *DAX1* on Xp21.3–21.2 is downregulated with testis differentiation but persists in the developing ovary. It may interact with SF-1 and antagonize the WT1 interaction to repress antimüllerian hormone expression, permitting development of the uterus and fallopian tubes. Increased expression of DAX1 in XY individuals with a duplication of Xp21 results in a female phenotype. WNT4, a cysteine-rich glycoprotein that functions as an extracellular signaling factor, serves to upregulate DAX1. If WNT4 is overexpressed, excessive DAX1 is produced, and a female phenotype results in XY individuals. In addition, WNT4 may suppress the growth of Leydig cells in the differentiating gonad through increased DAX1 and its antagonism of SRY. The lack of Leydig cells prevents the secretion of testosterone, which results in lack of stabilization of the wolffian ducts and failure of development of internal male genitalia.

GATA transcription factors are critical in continued reproductive development and function. GATA4, the same factor involved in cardiac septation, may be involved in ovarian folliculogenesis and the maintenance of granulosa cells. It is also expressed in Sertoli cells and may play a role in androgen steroidogenesis. Enzymes involved in the biosynthesis of testosterone are all necessary for the normal masculinization of external genitalia in XY individuals, and deficiencies result in ambiguous genitalia. However, excessive production of testosterone may result in masculinization of the XX individual's female genitalia, as discussed in 21-hydroxylase deficiency (see Chapter 7).

Normal androgen steroidogenesis and differentiation of male genitalia continue with transformation of testosterone to dihydrotestosterone by 5α-reductase type 2, normally expressed in fetal genital skin and the urogenital sinus. XY males homozygous for loss-of-function mutations in 5α-reductase type 2 have ambiguous genitalia at birth, including perineal hypospadias and a blind perineal pouch (pseudovaginal perineoscrotal hypospadias), and they develop masculinization at puberty when 5α-reductase type 1 normally begins to be synthesized. This delayed masculinization is an important consideration in the decision whether an individual should be reared as a female or a male.

Dihydrotestosterone exerts its influence on the cell through interaction with the androgen receptor (AR gene on Xq11-q12) and causes the androgen receptor to translocate to the nucleus, where it functions with other regulatory proteins in transcription control through the promoter region of a target gene. Loss-of-function mutations in AR produce complete androgen insensitivity in which affected XY males have female external genitalia, female breast development, a blind vagina, absent uterus and ovaries, and the presence of abdominal or inguinal testes. (Androgen insensitivity syndrome was historically referred to as testicular feminization, which does not accurately reflect the pathophysiology and may be offensive to patients and families.) Individuals with mutations that result in decreased expression of the androgen receptor have partial androgen insensitivity, or Reifenstein syndrome, with hypospadias, micropenis, gynecomastia, and azoospermia but with the presence of germ cells.

Features of mild androgen insensitivity are found in Kennedy spinal and bulbar muscular atrophy, but the phenotype does not present until puberty. Normal male external genitalia are present, and gynecomastia may develop at puberty along with sparse facial and body hair and impotence. Muscle fasciculations and weakness are typically noticed after 40 years of age. A polyglutamine tract in the coding region of exon 1 of AR normally has 10–33 CAG repeats. Expansion to more than 40 repeats is associated with the Kennedy phenotype.

ETHICS Stem Cells and Cloning

Many parts of the human genome are inactivated after embryonic development, making difficult the study of developmental biology in individuals born with congenital malformations. Investigators believe that these embryonically active genes have potential in regenerative medicine, which involves tissue engineering and other techniques aimed at repairing damaged or diseased tissues and organs. Some disorders, especially neuromuscular disorders such as Alzheimer disease and Parkinson disease, are particularly resistant to standard medical interventions because of the degeneration of cells of the nervous system.

Investigators wish to study the embryonically active genes found in totipotent stem cells to explore new avenues of therapy for these difficult disorders. However, these

ETHICS   Stem Cells and Cloning *(continued)*

embryonic stem cells have the potential for differentiation into a living human. Some individuals believe the following:

- The manipulation and study of embryonic stem cells will prevent a human life.
- Pregnancies will be terminated for the express purpose of retrieving embryonic stem cells.
- Manipulation of totipotent stem cells may result in eugenics, including engineering of humans with desired traits.

Pluripotent and multipotent stem cells that lack the ability to differentiate into a complete embryo may also be valuable in the investigation, but with our limited knowledge, they may have differentiated beyond the critical point of gene expression.

The term *cloning* has been used by molecular geneticists to describe creation of a copy of a gene for study. Recently the term has been used by the public to describe the emotionally charged area of **reproductive cloning,** in which the nucleus from an adult somatic cell is used to create offspring. The somatic cell nuclear transfer method of cloning was first accomplished in 1997 in sheep. A mammary cell nucleus from an adult white-faced ewe was transferred to the cytoplasm of another sheep ovum and placed in the uterus of a black-faced ewe. After 277 nuclear transfer attempts, which resulted in 29 viable embryos and one fetus, Dolly, a white-faced lamb, was born. The nuclear transfer technique has been used in livestock. Although the methods have become more efficient, fewer than 4% of embryos become viable offspring. In addition, unusually large offspring have been born to cattle or sheep following implantation of embryos manipulated by nuclear transfer; this is known as large-offspring syndrome.

Cloning has not yet been accomplished successfully in apes or humans in a process open to scientific scrutiny. Overgrowth syndromes (e.g., Beckwith-Wiedemann syndrome and insulin-like growth factor II) have been reported in humans through chromosomal abnormalities or genetic mutations, frequently involving imprinted genes. These overgrowth syndromes have some of the same features as large-offspring syndrome, including changes in organ and tissue development and placental anomalies. Therefore, large-offspring syndrome is hypothesized to be due to effects on imprinted genes, which may be particularly vulnerable to the imbalances in epigenetic modification that normally occur during gametogenesis. Concern has been raised that clones generated from transfer of an adult nucleus may have a shortened life expectancy due to telomeric shortening, but this has not been found to be the case.

Therapeutic cloning involves nuclear transfer cloning to extract pluripotent embryonic stem cells to provide a culture source of cells for regenerative medicine studies. The therapeutic potential of adult stem cells is much lower than that of embryonic stem cells because of limitations in the ability to manipulate the adult stem cells and loss of ability to differentiate into other cell and tissue types. Research to determine whether a mature cell can be induced to revert to the gene expression profile of an embryonic stem cell, alleviating the need to use human oocytes, is under way.

The views of a particular individual about stem cells and cloning frequently parallel his or her views about pregnancy termination, although those who are not in favor of abortion but who have family members affected with neurodegenerative disorders

(continues)

ETHICS   Stem Cells and Cloning (continued)

such as Parkinson disease and Huntington disease may advocate stem cell research or therapeutic cloning. Human reproductive cloning is considered to be excessively risky because of the unresolved issues of the disruption to imprinting and the increased risk of anomalies. Reproductive cloning has often been portrayed in science fiction as a method to obtain an exact copy of a person with replications of behavior and knowledge as well as physical traits. This view ignores the contributions of prenatal and postnatal environments on the developing individual. Compare this view to the natural occurrence of monozygotic twins, who share the same uterus and early childhood upbringing yet develop their own personalities and thoughts. A reproductive clone reared in a different uterus, years later, and exposed to a completely different childhood environment might have DNA identical to the original nuclear donor but would be his or her own person.

Even with the separation of science fiction from reality, a slippery slope runs between therapeutic cloning and reproductive cloning. Do the ends justify the means? Or will a Pandora's box be irreversibly opened?

USMLE-Style Questions

1. The Pierre-Robin anomaly is a combination of **U**-shaped cleft palate, micrognathia (small jaw), and posterior displacement of the tongue, which results from a failure of the tongue to drop from the superior nasopharynx in time for the palatal shelves to close. Which of the following terms best describes this anomaly?
   a. Deformation
   b. Disruption
   c. Malformation
   d. Sequence

2. An infant is born with an isolated ventricular septal defect. Which of the following terms best describes this anomaly?
   a. Deformation
   b. Disruption
   c. Malformation
   d. Sequence

3. An infant is born with ambiguous genitalia and a 46,XY karyotype. The child has an elevated testosterone level and no evidence of any uterus or fallopian tubes. Testes are present in the upper inguinal canal. At which point in sexual differentiation is the defect likely to have occurred?
   a. Heterozygous mutation in the *SRY* gene
   b. Lack of anti-müllerian hormone
   c. Lack of conversion of testosterone to dihydrotestosterone
   d. Total lack of the androgen receptor

SUGGESTED READINGS

Goodman FR. Congenital abnormalities of body patterning: embryology revisited. Lancet 2003;362:651–662.

Yagi H, Furutani Y, Hamada H, et al. Role of TBX1 in human del22q11.2 syndrome. Lancet 2003;362:1366–1373. *Provided proof of involvement of TBX1 in human disorders.*

Packham EA, Brook JD. T-box genes in human disorders. Hum Mol Genet 2003;12 Spec No 1:R37–44. *Good review of human disorders but written before Yagi et al.*

Baldini A. DiGeorge syndrome: the use of model organisms to dissect complex genetics. Hum Mol Genet 2002;11(20):2363–2369. *Good review of Tbx1 in mouse development.*

Garg V, Kathiriya IS, Barnes R, et al. GATA4 mutations cause human congenital heart defects and reveal an interaction with TBX5. Nature 2003;424:443–447.

MacLaughlin DT, Donahoe PK. Sex determination and differentiation. N Engl J Med 2004;350:367–378. *Good figures and diagrams.*

Hochedlinger K, Jaenisch R. Nuclear transplantation, embryonic stem cells, and the potential for cell therapy. N Engl J Med 2003;349:275–286.

WEB RESOURCES

http://www.med.unc.edu/embryo_images/
Embryo Images: normal and abnormal mammalian development. A tutorial that uses scanning electron micrographs as the primary resource to teach mammalian embryology. Beautiful images provide extensive surface detail.

http://embryo.soad.umich.edu/
The Multi-Dimensional Human Embryo. A collaboration funded by the National Institute of Child Health and Human Development to produce and make available over the internet a three-dimensional image reference of the human embryo based on magnetic resonance imaging.

http://www.genetests.org/
An excellent review on androgen insensitivity.

http://www.guideline.gov/summary/summary.aspx?doc_id=2770
National Guideline Clearinghouse. Evaluation of the newborn with developmental anomalies of the external genitalia. American Academy of Pediatrics, Committee on Genetics.

Individualized Medicine

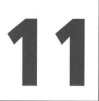
PHARMACOGENOMICS	INDIVIDUALIZED DRUG THERAPIES
Cytochrome P450 Family and Diversity	DISEASE SUSCEPTIBILITY
Gene Expression Microarrays	USMLE-STYLE QUESTIONS

In the clinic, rather than making diagnoses by goodness of fit of phenotypic features to a mythical classic case, we increasingly rely on precise molecular assays. As a consequence, we provide our patients and their families more accurate diagnosis and prognosis, together with more informed and effective management.

DAVID VALLE
2003 Presidential Address to the American Society of Human Genetics

In the preclinical years, much of the medical student's time is spent learning about classic presentations of disease, only to be told in the clinical years that only about 15 to 30% of disease is classic. The art of medicine consists of an intuitive approach to the patient that looks at the individual as a whole—a complex system of complex systems. Evidence-based medicine works well when the rules of a system are understood, but it breaks down when no study has yet been conducted to deal with the individual patient's complexities and exceptions to the rules. The future of medicine lies in **individualized medicine,** or personalized medicine, in which molecular evidence assists the art of medicine and combines numerous bits of evidence to tailor a therapeutic regimen to individual patients. Rather than having a one-size-fits -all clinical practice guideline, the molecular evidence permits individualized practice guidelines.

No two people are exactly alike. Even monozygotic twins have acquired their own specific somatic genetic mutations and psychological experiences. The Human Genome Project and the study of complex diseases have contributed to our knowledge of the individuality of each person, showing that interactions among polymorphisms and variations within the range of "normal" foster different reactions to events at the cellular level. Consider the different ways that individuals respond to the sights, sounds, smells, and tastes within their environment and the genetic variation that underlies their response. It is estimated that more than 75% of some classes of proteins may be polymorphic at the amino acid sequence level. Single-nucleotide polymorphisms (SNPs), alternative splicing, and epigenetics all have the potential to affect expression of genetic alleles. The effects on single genes have a cumulative impact on the systems within which the genes operate, and the larger networks with which the first system interacts—a complex web that is difficult to fathom.

We are just beginning to implement a rudimentary form of individualized medicine. Pharmacogenomics considers the effects of genetic polymorphisms on drug metabolism, response, and toxicity. The use of gene expression microarrays for individual tumors is an investigational tool used to tailor the appropriate cancer chemotherapy, the first area of designer drug therapies to become available. We are beginning to understand genetic variation and susceptibility to infectious diseases, such as human immunodeficiency virus (HIV). Advances in rapid analysis and bioinformatics are necessary before these techniques are widely available

149

and affordable. Individualized medicine is in its infancy but has the potential to incite a new revolution in health care. Unfortunately, individualized medicine also has the potential to create a new form of discrimination through genomic profiling of population groups.

PHARMACOGENOMICS

Since the 1950s, inheritance has been known to play a role in drug metabolism. **Pharmacogenetics** is the study of the role of inheritance in individual variation in drug metabolism phenotypes, such as fast or slow acetylators of isoniazid, pseudocholinesterase or butyrylcholinesterase deficiency (inability to hydrolyze succinylcholine), or the diversity of the cytochrome P450 enzyme system. **Pharmacogenomics,** the influence of variations in DNA sequences on the effect of drugs, plays a role as genomic sequence data become increasingly available. Drug metabolism phenotypes are being directly correlated with genetic polymorphisms found in drug metabolism enzymes. For most purposes, the terms pharmacogenetics and pharmacogenomics may be used interchangeably.

Known differences in drug response and reaction result from the effects of drug interactions, age, gender, and coexisting disease, but genetics may account for 20 to 95% of the known variability. The many families of drug reaction proteins in humans all have genetic variants. They represent phase I metabolism reactions (oxidation, reduction, and hydrolysis), phase II metabolism reactions (acetylation, glucuronidation, sulfation, and methylation), drug transporters, and drug receptors. Most of the variability occurs through the more than 1 million SNPs that have been identified in the human genome. (*CYP2C9*, a member of the phase I cytochrome P450 family, was discussed in Chapter 4 as an example of clinically relevant SNPs.) Some unique SNPs have been identified in some extreme cases, but most drug effects are moderated by several interacting gene products. The polygenic genotypes interact to produce the drug response phenotype, which includes efficacy and toxicity.

Pharmacogenomics provides additional information on variations in the drug response

observed in individuals within and among ethnic groups. The prevalence of SNPs varies widely among ethnic groups and plays an important role in the differences in response to therapeutic regimens. The introduction of pharmacogenomics into clinical trials and the required inclusion of diverse groups of people will increase the likelihood of safer and more effective therapies for all individuals.

Cytochrome P450 Family and Diversity

The CYP3A subfamily of the cytochrome P450 family illustrates the issue of diversity. The most important drug-metabolizing enzymes in humans, CYP3A enzymes are abundantly expressed in the liver and are responsible for oxidative metabolism of 50 to 60% of clinically used drugs. CYP3A activity consists of the sum of the activity of all subfamily members. *CYP3A4* and *CYP3A5* are the most heavily expressed, are induced by a wide variety of drugs, and share 85% homology. Induction of gene expression by one drug may increase the amount of available enzyme, which increases the rate of metabolism of all drugs affected by the CYP3A family. The over-the-counter herbal product St John's wort is also capable of inducing CYP3A4, which may result in reduced clinical effectiveness or a requirement of increased dosage for a number of prescription medications.

CYP3A4 has very few variants, and those have limited functional significance. However, *CYP3A5* has a number of polymorphisms and highly variable expression in humans. SNPs in the *CYP3A5*3* and *CYP3A5*6* alleles cause alternative splicing and protein truncation, with the absence of CYP3A5 in some individuals. The presence of the *CYP3A5*1* allele results in the expression of large amounts of CYP3A5. Relatively high levels of CYP3A5 are expressed by an estimated 30% of whites, 30% of Japanese, 30% of Mexicans, 40% of Chinese, and more than 50% of African Americans, southeast Asians, Pacific Islanders, and southwestern Native Americans. CYP3A5 may be the most important genetic contributor to individual and racial differences in responses to many medications because of differences in

CYP3A-dependent drug clearance. Nonwhite persons are likely to have higher clearance of drugs and are less likely to have drug toxicities than whites.

The CYP2D family, specifically CYP2D6, is important in the metabolism of more than 30 drugs and environmental chemicals, including as many as 20% of commonly prescribed medications. CYP2D6 hydroxylates many drugs, such as the β-blockers propranolol and metoprolol, the tricyclic antidepressants nortriptyline and amitriptyline, and the antipsychotic haloperidol. CYP2D6 activity ranges from absent to "poor hydroxylator" to the "ultrarapid hydroxylator." Several alleles have been found to contribute to the poor-hydroxylator phenotype, which has a 9% prevalence in the United Kingdom but a 30% prevalence in Chinese Hong Kong. Chinese people have a greater sensitivity to the β-blocking effects of propranolol. The ultrarapid metabolizer phenotype is associated with amplification of a *CYP2D6* allele; some individuals have as many as 12 or 13 copies. Individuals with multiple copies of *CYP2D6* are found in different proportions in various populations: 1 to 2% in Chinese, Germans, and black Zimbabweans; 20% in Saudis; and 29% in Ethiopians. Responses to antidepressant drug therapy are known to vary widely among individuals, which may be explained by the range of response phenotypes.

The same variability that exists in drug metabolism enzymes may also be found in drug transporters and drug receptors. The P-glycoprotein, encoded by *ABCB1* on 7q21.1, is a transmembrane drug transporter which extrudes a variety of drugs from the cytoplasm across the plasma membrane. Its natural substrates are digitalis-like substances. Individuals with a homozygous C3435T polymorphism have significantly lower *ABCB1* expression, which results in high plasma levels of digoxin. *ABCB1* is also induced by normally occurring genes. Paclitaxel (Taxol) induces a nuclear receptor which activates *CYP3A4* expression as well as *ABCB1*. The related compound docetaxel (Taxotere) does not induce the nuclear receptor and has superior pharmacokinetic properties. When overexpressed through amplification or creation of a fusion gene in cancer cells, multidrug resistance develops.

Gene Expression Microarrays

Relatively few clinical tests permit the practical use of pharmacogenomics. The advent of microarray technology may facilitate its incorporation into mainstream medicine by permitting clinicians to select medications and drug doses for individual patients. The time needed for titration of the optimal dose may be reduced, because it will be possible to determine who needs to start at a lower dose because of reduced drug metabolism and who needs to start at a much higher dose because of rapid metabolism. A person's genotype for each gene must be determined only once because of the low likelihood of somatic mutations.

Gene expression microarrays are used to study the types and quantity of mRNA produced by a cell. In review, a given mRNA molecule hybridizes specifically to the DNA template from which it originated. An array containing many DNA samples can be constructed, and in one experiment, the expression levels of hundreds or thousands of genes can be measured by the amount of mRNA binding to the spots on the microarray. The DNA microarray is usually a solid object the size of a large postage stamp or microscope slide. The DNA fragments are synthesized directly onto the solid frame in a known grid pattern.

Microarray technology must be improved to be suitable for use in a clinical facility rather than in a research environment. Complex statistical and computational tools are required to determine patterns in the raw microarray data of thousands of genes. Currently it costs about $1000 to test a single tissue sample, without considering the necessary repetitions for quality control and verification required by the Clinical Laboratories Improvement Act or the special expertise necessary to interpret the data.

INDIVIDUALIZED DRUG THERAPIES

The diagnosis and prognosis of most human cancers has relied heavily on descriptive histopathological data. Increasingly, molecular testing is used to provide a more precise description of cancer behavior and characteristics. DNA microarray technology has been used widely in cancer research and has identified unique profiles of cancers that are otherwise indistinguishable under the microscope. Designer drugs that interact with very specific receptors and cell types have been created, allowing a reduction in toxicity of the therapeutic regimen. Historically, the approach to cancer chemotherapy has been to poison the patient in a controlled fashion to kill as many rapidly growing cells as possible, but this may bring the patient close to death. It is the equivalent of using a sledge hammer to drive in a nail. Individualized drug therapies permit selection of a hammer of appropriate size. The expectation is that individualized medicine will increase treatment efficacy while decreasing toxicity and controlling health care expenses.

In the near future, it may be financially feasible to use microarray technology to perform diagnostic gene expression profiles of tumors. This assumes that small sets of genes can be identified, which will facilitate diagnostic distinctions among tumors that are difficult to distinguish by normal histopathology. Investigators have found a set of six genes whose expression predicts survival in individuals with diffuse large B-cell lymphoma. Three of the genes (LMO2, BCL6, FN1) are associated with longer overall survival, and three (CCND2, SCYA3, BCL2) are associated with shorter overall survival (Table 11.1). The relative contributions of each gene were used to calculate a mortality predictor score, which was validated in individuals with diffuse large B-cell lymphoma. This type of gene expression profile is more economical to pursue than a genome-wide scan of gene expression.

DISEASE SUSCEPTIBILITY

The interplay of genetic code, epigenetics, genetic control mechanisms, and environmental factors is a hallmark of complex diseases (see Chapter 9). Different diseases are caused by varying contributions of the factors. Infectious diseases have been interpreted to be almost exclusively environmental. However, an individual's genetic background may also determine the initial susceptibility to the microbial agent and the response to routine antibiotic therapy.

The entry of the HIV-1 virus into human cells is a complex process. Some strains of the HIV-1 envelope glycoprotein gp120 interact consecutively with T-cell surface antigen CD4 and the CCR5 surface receptor, a G protein-coupled receptor that activates multiple intracellular signaling pathways (Fig. 11.1). Other strains interact with the CXCR4 surface receptor. Amino acids 2 to 18 of the CCR5 amino terminal domain form the gp120 binding site. Infection of human T cells results in their loss, and infection of macrophages produces a viral reservoir. HIV-1 also interacts with receptors of neurons and astrocytes. Agents that serve as either CCR5 or CXCR4 receptor antagonists are being developed to limit HIV-1 infectivity.

Some individuals have been noted to have slow disease progression from HIV-1 infection to development of AIDS. These people are likely to be heterozygous for a CCR5 allele with a 32-bp deletion (Δ32), which results in a frameshift mutation after amino acid 174, inclusion of 31 novel amino acids, and protein truncation at codon 206. The severely truncated protein cannot be detected on the cell surface and lacks the regions involved in G-protein coupling and signal transduction. Individuals who are homozygous for the Δ32 allele are incapable of becoming infected with the CCR5-specific strains of HIV-1 and have no known phenotypic abnormalities. The Δ32 allele is present primarily in populations of European descent, and the frequency pattern follows a north-south gradient (highest in Finnish [16%] and lowest in Sardinians [4%]). It is thought that the Δ32 allele originated from a single mutation that probably arose a few thousand years ago in northeastern Europe. It has been found at frequencies of 2 to 5% in individuals in the Middle East and India but is virtually absent among native African, American Indian, and East Asian ethnic groups.

TABLE 11.1 GENES IN GENE EXPRESSION PROFILE USED TO PREDICT SURVIVAL IN DIFFUSE LARGE B-CELL LYMPHOMA

GENE AND LOCATION	NAME	NORMAL GENE FUNCTION	FUNCTION IF MUTATED	IMPACT OF EXPRESSION ON SURVIVAL
LMO2 11p13	LIM domain only 2	Hematopoietic progenitors and erythropoiesis; bridging molecule in transcription factor complexes	Oncogene in T-cell leukemias	Longer
BCL6 3q27	B cell lymphoma 6	Transcriptional repressor needed for cells to have a germinal center fate and move away from plasma cell fate	Deregulated in fusion genes in diffuse large cell lymphomas and follicular lymphomas	Longer
FN1 2q34	Fibronectin 1	Cell surface glycoprotein; cellular adhesion	Ehlers-Danlos syndrome with platelet dysfunction	Longer
CCND2 12p13	Cyclin D2	G1 phase of cell cycle; promotes progression to DNA synthesis	Unknown	Shorter
SCYA3 17q11-q12	Small inducible cytokine A3	Early G0/G1 switch gene; recruitment and activation of neutrophils	Unknown	Shorter
BCL2 18q21.3	B cell/CLL lymphoma 2	Inhibitor of apoptosis	Deregulated fusion gene in follicular lymphoma and chronic lymphocytic leukemia	Shorter

Data from Lossos IS, Czerwinski DK, Alizadeh AA, et al. Prediction of survival in diffuse large-B-cell lymphoma based on the expression of six genes. N Engl J Med 2004;350:1828–1837.

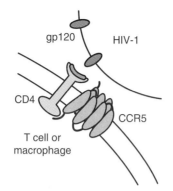

FIGURE 11.1 Entry of the human immunodeficiency virus type 1 (HIV-1) virus into its human host cell requires interaction between an HIV cell surface glycoprotein (gp120), the CD4 antigen and CCR5 (CC cytokine family receptor) or CXCR4 (CXC cytokine family receptor).

ETHICS Genetic Discrimination in the Future

The 1997 science fiction movie *GATTACA* shows a future in which it is possible not only to perform a complete and rapid genetic analysis of any individual but to genetically engineer infants with desired characteristics. Only "valid" genetically engineered individuals have places of significance in society. Children born naturally, without genetic engineering, are considered "in-valid" and are permitted only in menial jobs. The lead character is an "in-valid" who masquerades as a "valid" so he can have a career as a space traveler rather than as a custodian. He states, "We now have discrimination down to a science." The title itself, *GATTACA,* is a heptanucleotide DNA sequence.

We have discussed how new technologies and knowledge in medical genetics will lead to a new era of individualized molecular medicine resulting in more-effective and less-toxic therapy. Genetic information may also be misused. It can be used to discriminate against people in employment or health insurance. Each one of us probably has six or more mutations in our genome, which may predispose us to disease, so we all would be classified as "in-valid" in the *GATTACA* world.

Surveys have indicated that 75 to 85% of people would not want their insurance company or employer to have access to their genetic code. The Ethical, Legal and Social Implications (ELSI) Working Group of the Human Genome Project recommended in 1993 that health insurers be prohibited from using genetic information or a request for genetic services to deny or limit health insurance coverage or to establish differential premium rates and from obtaining an individual's genetic information without that individual's written authorization.

The Health Insurance Portability and Accountability Act (HIPAA) of 1996 provided the first federal protection against genetic discrimination in health insurance. The act prohibits health insurers from excluding individuals from group coverage because of genetic predisposition to diseases. The law specifically states that genetic information without a current diagnosis of disease does not constitute a preexisting condition. However, HIPAA does not prevent health insurers from charging a higher premium or from collecting or disclosing genetic information. In 2000, President Bill Clinton issued an executive order prohibiting federal agencies from obtaining genetic information

ETHICS   **Genetic Discrimination in the Future** *(continued)*

and from using it in hiring and promotion decisions. The President said, "We must not allow advances in genetics to become the basis of discrimination against any individual or any group. We must never allow these discoveries to change the basic belief upon which our government, our society, and our system of ethics is founded—that all of us are created equal, entitled to equal treatment under the law."

No additional federal legislation has been enacted. However, most states have enacted legislation protecting against genetic discrimination by health insurers or employers.

USMLE-Style Questions

1. *CYP3A5* functions using which of the following mechanisms?
   a. Acetylation of antimicrobials
   b. Antagonism of cell surface receptor
   c. Hydroxylation of tricyclic antidepressants
   d. Inhibition of hepatic metabolism
   e. Oxidation of therapeutic agents
2. *CYP2D6* activity is sharply increased in some individuals of Ethiopian or Saudi ancestry. Which of the following is the cause?
   a. Amplification of the gene
   b. Anticipation within the genome
   c. Gain-of-function missense mutations
   d. Induction of hepatic enzymes
   e. Protein truncation due to frameshift mutations

SUGGESTED READINGS

Valle D. Genetics, individuality, and medicine in the 21st century. Am J Hum Genet 2004;74:374–381.

Weinshilboum R. Inheritance and drug response. N Engl J Med 2003;348:529–537.

Evans WE, McLeod HL. Pharmacogenomics: drug disposition, drug targets, and side effects. N Engl J Med 2003;348:538–549.

Ramaswamy S. Translating cancer genomics into clinical oncology. N Engl J Med 2004; 350: 1814–1816.

Lossos IS, Czerwinski DK, Alizadeh AA, et al. Prediction of survival in diffuse large-B-cell lymphoma based on the expression of six genes. N Engl J Med 2004;350:1828–1837.

WEB RESOURCES

http://www.ornl.gov/sci/techresources/Human_Genome/medicine/pharma.shtml
   Pharmacogenomics information from the U.S. Department of Energy Office of Science, Office of Biological and Environmental Research, Human Genome Program.

http://www.ncbi.nlm.nih.gov/About/primer/pharm.html
   A science primer on pharmacogenomics from the National Center for Biotechnology Information.

http://www.ncbi.nlm.nih.gov/About/primer/microarrays.html
   A science primer on DNA microarrays from the National Center for Biotechnology Information. This is an excellent and understandable review of microarray technology.

http://www.genome.gov/10002328
   Genetic discrimination fact sheet from the National Human Genome Research Institute.

Gene Therapy

VIRAL VECTORS
    Retroviral Vectors
    Adenoviral Vectors
    Adeno-Associated Viral Vectors

NONVIRAL VECTORS
USMLE-STYLE QUESTIONS

In the 1970s, advances in molecular genetic technology fueled hope that it would be possible in the near future to correct a single-gene disorder simply by placing the normal gene into body cells. Ethical concerns stemming from eugenics steered interventions into altering somatic cells to avoid altering germ cells. Initially, scientists seriously underestimated the difficulties that would have to be overcome, and continued technical problems have caused gene therapy to remain as a hypothetical treatment modality rather than a practical one. As steps have been taken to overcome the technical problems, new side effects of gene therapy have been exposed, making people cautious. In the past, once a gene was identified and the sequence delineated, scientists proclaimed that gene therapy for the disorder would occur in the very near future. No longer do most scientists hurry to make this announcement, but the lay press continues to stress it.

In March 1998, the U.S. Food and Drug Administration defined **gene therapy** as a medical intervention based on modification of the genetic material of living cells through either in vivo therapy given directly to a patient or ex vivo therapy, manipulation of cells outside the patient for subsequent administration. The latter is a form of **somatic cell therapy,** the ex vivo manipulation and subsequent reintroduction of somatic cells into an individual.

VIRAL VECTORS

One of the most difficult challenges has been the task of delivering the genetic material to the cells that require it. Hematopoietic cells may be removed from the person, manipulated ex vivo, and returned with minimal difficulty, but this has the potential to affect only disorders expressed in hematopoietic cell lines, such as immune deficiencies and hemoglobinopathies. For disorders which involve less accessible cell types, such as pulmonary or hepatic cells, delivery has been a much greater obstacle.

Most forms of gene therapy use viral delivery mechanisms, because viruses naturally function to insert their genetic material into the host cell for incorporation, replication, and release leading to infection of other cells. Retrovirus and adenovirus vectors have been the most commonly used vectors in gene transfer trials. The viruses are altered to eliminate the propagation of the viral DNA but to maintain the ability of the virus to insert DNA into the host cells.

Retroviral Vectors

Retroviral vectors are used in gene therapy because retroviruses are RNA viruses that have reverse transcriptase to transcribe the RNA into DNA, which is then inserted stably into the host genome. One of the first gene therapy trials began in the early 1990s, using retroviruses in an ex vivo somatic cell treatment of hematopoietic cells. Deficiency of adenosine deaminase (*ADA* on 20q13.11) results in a severe combined immunodeficiency (SCID) with dysfunction of both B- and T-cell lymphocytes, resulting in decreased cellular immunity and decreased production of immunoglobulins. ADA deficiency is responsible for approximately half of autosomal recessive forms of SCID. The gene therapy trials involved repeated retrovirus-mediated transfer of the *ADA* gene into stimulated peripheral blood lymphocytes of two children. It is generally agreed that these initial trials were unsuccessful in correcting the immune deficiency in ADA-SCID, but one of the patients still shows more than 15% of peripheral lymphocytes with the inserted gene and an ADA activity approximately 25% of normal. Results of a more recent and more clinically successful trial using updated methodology were announced in 2002.

X-linked severe combined immunodeficiency (X-SCID) is another form of combined cellular and humoral immunodeficiency resulting from a lack of T lymphocytes and natural killer lymphocytes and nonfunction of B lymphocytes. Boys with X-SCID typically develop symptoms between 3 and 6 months of age, with failure to thrive, oral or diaper candidiasis, absent tonsils and lymph nodes, recurrent persistent infections, and infections with opportunistic organisms. Life expectancy is significantly shortened. Affected boys have a mutation in the interleukin-2 receptor-γ gene (*IL2RG*) at Xq13.1. The interleukin-2 lymphokine interacts with its receptors and affects the growth and differentiation of common lymphoid progenitors into T cells, B cells, and natural killer cells, as well as the growth and differentiation of glioma cells and monocytes. High-affinity interleukin-2 receptors consist of α-β-γ heterotrimers, and intermediate-affinity receptors consist of β-γ heterodimers. In X-SCID, the combined immunodeficiency results from failure of normal lymphopoiesis. In 2002, it was shown that in vitro manipulation of hematopoietic stem cells with retroviral insertion of *IL2RG* could result in normal immune function after return of the manipulated cells to individuals affected with X-SCID. In the French X-SCID gene therapy trial, recovery of immune function in 9 of 10 boys has lasted several years, and they are being followed to determine whether this continues.

Retroviruses insert their DNA into host DNA on active genes near gene promoters, and investigators are not yet able to control the specific insertion site. Retroviral insertions may also enhance the expression of host cell genes surrounding the insertion site (**insertional mutagenesis**), causing unplanned side effects. Retroviral insertional mutagenesis in mice has been associated with leukemia and has permitted the identification of leukemia oncogenes. Unfortunately, 2 of the 10 boys in the X-SCID gene therapy trial developed T-cell acute lymphoblastic leukemia (ALL) several years after the hematopoietic cells altered by retroviruses began to grow in their bone marrow. In these boys, the retroviral integration site was very close to or within the T-cell oncogene *LMO2* (see Table 11.1), causing aberrant expression of *LMO2*, which is also activated in chromosomal translocations typically found in T-cell ALL. Translocations occur upstream of one or both of the *LMO2* promoters. In both boys with leukemia, the retroviral insertion site, which was near one or both of the promoter sites, resulted in enhanced expression of *LMO2*. *LMO2* is expressed early in hematopoiesis. Therefore, it is active in hematopoietic stem cells and so is an ideal target for retroviral insertion. One of the affected boys developed leukemia immediately after a varicella zoster infection, and the other affected boy had an acquired mutation in another T-cell oncogene, *TAL1* (*T*-cell *a*cute *l*ymphocytic leukemia-1), suggesting that additional DNA changes were needed for the actual development of leukemia. A third boy, who has not developed leukemia, also has a retroviral insertion site in the *LMO2* region.

Adenoviral Vectors

Adenoviral vectors are used in 25 to 30% of gene therapy trials, ranking second only to retroviral vectors. Adenoviruses are a group of linear double-stranded DNA-containing viruses that are primarily associated with upper and lower respiratory disease. Able to infect both dividing and nondividing cells, adenoviruses do not integrate into the host cell genome. Gene expression following adenoviral gene transfer is short lived. Because of their association with upper respiratory disease, adenoviral vectors were used initially in gene therapy trials for cystic fibrosis beginning in 1993. The genetic abnormality in cystic fibrosis is not expressed in the readily accessible hematopoietic cells; therefore, the vector must be able to reach the appropriate cells. In trials, adenovirus infectivity of respiratory epithelial cells was lower than expected. Infectivity was altered by the normal protective function of the airway epithelium—prevention of uptake of foreign materials through extracellular barriers such as mucus, the glycocalyx (extracellular coating of glycoproteins and proteoglycans), and mucociliary clearance. The receptors for adenoviruses lie on the basolateral membrane of the cells rather than the more accessible apical membrane. In addition, transfected cells were shed within a few months, which implied that the lung repopulating stem cells were not receiving the inserted gene. Gene therapy for treatment of cystic fibrosis therefore requires repeated administrations of the transfer agents; this is a particular problem with adenovirus, because individuals develop an adaptive immunological response to the virus.

The immune response to adenovirus vectors is extremely complex, involves both innate and adaptive immune responses, and contributes heavily to toxicity associated with the vector. Deficiency of ornithine carbamoyltransferase (formerly known as ornithine transcarbamylase, or OTC) is an abnormality of the urea cycle. *OTC*, which is at Xp21.1, catalyzes the second step in the cycle. Boys with OTC deficiency accumulate ammonia and related metabolites in the first few days of life, with symptoms progressing from initial vomiting and sleepiness to eventual seizures and coma with resulting brain damage. The severity of the phenotype is determined by the level of enzyme expressed; some carrier females may demonstrate a mild phenotype when challenged with pregnancy, illness, or a high-protein diet. *OTC* is expressed primarily in the liver and small intestinal mucosa, which also presented challenges for vector delivery in gene therapy.

A clinical trial in partial OTC deficiency used hepatic artery infusions with increasing dosages of adenoviral vector particles. As the vector distributes in the blood, an initial response occurs within minutes and is attributed to an innate response without need for viral gene expression. The adenoviral vector interacts with reticuloendothelial cells and induces the release of proinflammatory cytokines. In addition, macrophages are targeted, leading to a systemic acquired immune response. This response may be lethal and can occur within days, with extensive endothelial damage and disseminated intravascular coagulopathy. In 1999, one patient died in the course of the clinical trial (discussed in the Ethics box). It is now known that toxicity may be reduced by pretreatment with anti-inflammatory agents such as steroids.

Targeted delivery of adenovirus in disorders that do not require repeated administration of adenovirus may prove to have much less vector-induced toxicity. Gene therapy to induce neovascularization of individuals with ischemic limb and heart disease has promise. Neovascularization is a complex series of events involved in the production of new blood vessels, which occurs as a natural compensatory process in individuals with coronary artery disease and peripheral vascular disease (Box 12.1). However, the natural process is frequently inadequate; clinical symptoms may occur, and surgical revascularization, such as coronary artery bypass, may be necessary. Therapeutic angiogenesis is the attempt to induce neovascularization by angiogenic agents delivered directly or via gene transfer. Although gene transfer has the potential benefit of persistent expression after a single administration, it carries the risk of vector-induced inflammation, transfer to surrounding unaffected cells, and lack of gene regulation with uncontrolled expression. Another challenge is that no single gene is likely to provide sufficient neovascularization by itself.

Research is evaluating the effects of insertion of vasculogenesis factors on coronary artery disease. Endothelial cell growth factor, or fibroblast growth factor 1 (FGF1), is a modifier of endothelial cell migration and proliferation. Additional FGFs also influence endothelial cell growth and other types of embryological growth (see Fig. 10.3). A replication-defective

---

BOX 12.1

Processes Involved in Neovascularization

- Vasculogenesis
  — Formation of new blood vessels from embryonic pluripotent stem cells
  — Mobilizes endothelial progenitor cells from bone marrow in adults
- Angiogenesis
  — Capillary growth from enlarged venules
  — Capillaries proliferating in wound healing and at the border of myocardial infarctions
- Arteriogenesis
  — Formation of true collateral arteries with fully developed tunica media
  — Smooth muscle cell growth and proliferation, migration, and differentiation to a contractile phenotype

---

adenovirus containing the *FGF4* gene was injected once into the coronary artery of individuals with stable angina pectoris with no immediate adverse effects and no serious long-term effects. However, there was no significant increase in neovascularization. Vascular endothelial growth factor (VEGF) specifically acts on endothelial cells. Experiments in rats have shown decreased production of VEGF as the animals age, with enhanced production after adenoviral-mediated *VEGF* gene transfer. Intramyocardial delivery of the vector in pigs has produced a higher expression rate than did intracoronary artery delivery.

Adeno-Associated Viral Vectors

Adeno-associated viral (AAV) vectors, derived from a nonpathogenic single-strand DNA parvovirus, demonstrate lack of cytotoxic lymphocyte response. They require coinfection with a helper virus (adenovirus or herpesvirus)

to undergo productive infection, and they integrate preferentially into 19q13.3 of the human genome, facilitating longer gene expression. AAV can infect both nondividing and dividing cells. AAV2 has been used to transfer the *CFTR* gene in individuals with mild pulmonary disease and cystic fibrosis. Because of the decreased immune response to AAV, repeated doses are feasible, which facilitates pulmonary function somewhat without adverse effects.

Hemophilia caused by deficiencies in either factor VIII or factor IX requires lifelong therapy. Effective gene therapy requires sustained production of coagulation factor at therapeutic levels, which puts additional pressure on safety and prevention of an immune response to a vector. In addition, individuals who naturally have an absence of factor VIII or IX may develop an immune response to the newly generated protein, just as they may develop an immune response to administration of the synthetic protein product. Because of the need for long-term expression, retroviruses and AAV have been examined as vectors. AAV1 with factor IX has been injected into the skeletal muscle of mice and produced sustained levels above the therapeutic range, probably due to the number of myocytes effectively transfected. When AAV2 is used as the vector, expression rates in mice are only 1% of those produced with AAV1. Data also indicate that significant species differences occur in terms of the rate of cell infectivity and gene expression. Clinical trials with human subjects are in progress.

NONVIRAL VECTORS

Nonviral vectors produce a less severe immune response than virus-mediated gene therapy. However, extracellular DNA is recognized by the immune system of the host, particularly if unmethylated CpG regions are present, as is typical of bacterial plasmids holding the DNA to be transported.

Liposomes are artificial cationic single or laminar vesicles made from lipids that are constructed to form a nonimmunogenic complex with DNA capable of internalization into the cytoplasm of the cell through fusion with the cellular membrane. Once within the cytoplasm, the complex dissociates through normal intracellular metabolic processes, releasing the DNA within the cell. The particles are smaller than viral vectors, improving diffusion. However, entry into the nucleus is problematic, because peptides are used to signal active transport. **Peptide** gene carriers, which form a stable complex with DNA, have also been used. Specific peptide sequences assist in targeted delivery of genes in vivo and facilitate active transport through the nuclear pores. Biodegradable or thermosensitive polymers, which also are capable of forming complexes with DNA, have been developed. Most of the nonviral vector work has been conducted in rodents, and minimal information regarding its applicability to larger animals is available.

Naked DNA gene transfer has been used in clinical trials to treat peripheral arterial occlusion disease. Direct injection of plasmid DNA into skeletal muscle has been performed using either *VEGF* or *FGF1*. In the trial involving *FGF1*, no increase in FGF1 serum levels was apparent, but transcutaneous oxygen pressure improved, suggesting that localized expression of *FGF1* may be effective. Intravascular delivery into the limb with temporary occlusion with a blood pressure cuff may also permit more widespread delivery of the gene to the limb. Another potential use for naked DNA gene transfer is the development of a human immunodeficiency virus (HIV) vaccine. CD4 and CD8 T cells provide some limitation to HIV replication. Studies in nonhuman primates have found that CD8 immunity can be effectively induced by priming with naked plasmid DNA and then boosting immunity with recombinant viral vectors containing various parts of the HIV genome. Clinical trials using human subjects have begun.

ETHICS   The First Human Death from Gene Therapy

Severe deficiency of ornithine carbamoyltransferase (formerly known as ornithine transcarbamylase, or OTC) has a devastating phenotype. After beginning to eat, affected newborn boys develop lethargy and seizures shortly as a result of the protein load, and they become comatose within 3 days as a result of the hyperammonemia. The longer the exposure to elevated ammonia levels, the more severe the resulting brain damage. Treatment is possible but is frequently initiated after the damage has been done. At the University of Pennsylvania, scientists believed that OTC deficiency was an appropriate early target for a gene therapy trial. However, university bioethicists did not believe that newborn infants were appropriate subjects for this type of cutting-edge research, because parents of dying infants are so desperate for a cure that they are easily coerced into participating and incapable of giving true informed consent.

Instead, stable adult males with partial OTC deficiency or adult females with a mild phenotype were tested, with the consent of the National Urea Cycle Disorders Foundation. The researchers recruited 18 adults to receive an adenovirus vector *OTC* infusion into the hepatic artery to determine the maximum tolerated dose of vector. Six groups of three subjects were treated at increasingly high doses, a normal procedure for phase I clinical trials. Numerous mouse and primate studies preceded the human trial, with the data supporting continuation of the research. However, two rhesus monkeys given 20 times the planned peak human dose developed coagulopathy and liver dysfunction and died. No one had ever injected adenovirus directly into the hepatic artery in humans before, either.

Jesse Gelsinger, a 17-year-old boy, had partial OTC deficiency due to somatic mosaicism. After waiting until he was 18, he signed up for the clinical trial with the

(continues)

ETHICS **The First Human Death from Gene Therapy (*continued*)**

support of his family. After undergoing some screening laboratory studies, he was scheduled to be the second in the group of three to receive the highest dose of vector. After receiving his injection in September 1999, he became nauseated and developed a fever, just like four other subjects who received lower doses. However, the next morning, he was disoriented and jaundiced, with evidence of coagulopathy. He developed hyperammonemia, became comatose, and received dialysis. Despite extraordinary levels of intensive care, his condition worsened, and he developed multiple organ system failure. Brain death was declared, and life support was stopped.

Questions were raised about the adequacy and quality of the informed consent process and the failure of the university to report toxic side effects in the previous human subjects. Jesse's father stated that he was not informed about the deaths of the two monkeys or the reaction of the earlier patients. The National Institutes of Health asked gene therapy researchers all over the United States about adverse reactions and received reports of more than 650 reactions that had not been previously reported. Gene therapy trials throughout the country were put on hold.

Protection for patients is jeopardized by the interaction of many components, such as trade secrets, financial conflicts of interest due to the privatization of science, overloaded review committees, and patients' overwhelming desire for a cure. In Jesse's case, the U.S. Food and Drug Administration investigators charged the clinical researchers with the following:

- Inadequate informed consent
- Allowing Jesse to participate in the study even though his initial liver function studies did not meet the parameters for inclusion
- Failure to immediately notify the Food and Drug Administration of serious side effects in earlier patients
- Financial conflict of interest between a genetic technology company that contributed 25% of the institute's annual budget

The technology of gene therapy did not generate these research violations. They were incited by the pressure to produce results in a competitive field with corporate, rather than altruistic, intentions. As the Hippocratic oath states, "Do no harm."

USMLE-Style Questions

1. Gene therapy is being designed that would insert a gene into the host genome for extended duration of therapy. Which of the following vectors is most appropriate?
   a. Adeno-associated virus
   b. Adenovirus
   c. Liposome
   d. Naked DNA transfer
   e. Peptide package

2. A vector inserts its genetic load into the host genome near a promoter of an active-ly expressed gene. Which of the following vectors is known to function in this way?
   a. Adeno-associated virus
   b. Adenovirus
   c. Naked DNA transfer
   d. Parvovirus
   e. Retrovirus

SUGGESTED READINGS

Blaese RM, Culver KW, Miller AD, et al. T lymphocyte-directed gene therapy for ADA-SCID: initial trial results after 4 years. Science 1995;270:475–480.

Aiuti A, Slavin S, Aker M, et al. Correction of ADA-SCID by stem cell gene therapy combined with non-

myeloablative conditioning. Science 2002;296:
2410–2413.

Hacein-Bey-Abina S, Le Deist F, Carlier F, et al.
Sustained correction of X-linked severe combined
immunodeficiency by ex vivo gene therapy. 2002; N
Engl J Med 346:1185–1193.

Hacein-Bey-Abina S, von Kalle C, Schmidt M, et al. A
serious adverse event after successful gene therapy
for X-linked severe combined immunodeficiency. N
Engl J Med 2003;348:255–256.

McCormack MP, Rabbitts TH. Activation of the T-cell
oncogene *LMO2* after gene therapy for X-linked
severe combined immunodeficiency. N Engl J Med
2004;350:913–922.

Grines CL, Watkins MW, Helmer G, et al. Angiogenic
Gene Therapy (AGENT) trial in patients with
stable angina pectoris. Circulation 2002;105:
1291–1297.

Moss RB, Rodman D, Spencer LT, et al. Repeated
adeno-associated virus serotype 2 aerosol-mediated
cystic fibrosis transmembrane regulator gene transfer
to the lungs of patients with cystic fibrosis: a multi-
center, double-blind, placebo-controlled trial. Chest
2004;125:509–521.

WEB RESOURCES

http://www.nature.com/gt/progress_and_prospects.html
Gene Therapy Progress and Prospects. Each review
is written by leaders in the field, summarizes the last
two years of progress in a specific aspect of gene
therapy research, and highlights prospects for the
next two years.

http://www.genetests.org
Good review of X-linked severe combined immunodeficiency (X-SCID) and urea cycle disorders
(ornithine carbamoyltransferase deficiency).

http://www.clinicaltrials.gov
A service of the National Institutes of Health that
provides regularly updated information about feder-
ally and privately supported clinical research in
human volunteers. A good source for monitoring
clinical trials in gene therapy.

Answers to USMLE-Style Questions

CHAPTER 1

1. D. Positive eugenics encourages reproduction to produce desirable traits, such as intelligent medical students. Beneficence (A) implies helping the individual, and no evidence exists that having multiple children enhances the life of a medical student. Negative eugenics (B) implies discouraging reproduction by individuals with undesirable heritable traits, such as egocentric medical students, and is not stated by the parents in this scenario. The counseling provided by the parents is directive rather than nondirective (C).

2. B. The speaker discouraged the reproduction of immigrants he perceived as unfit; this is negative eugenics. Justice (A) implies equal access to health care and opportunities, a topic not addressed by this example. Individuals who are prevented from following individual rights through the practice of negative eugenics are not being shown a respect for autonomy (D).

CHAPTER 2

1. C. It is important to recognize the difference between mitosis, with its random alignment of chromosomes at the mitotic spindle, and meiosis, with the pairing of homologous chromosomes. Prophase is marked by activated cohesin and the binding together of the chromatids. Metaphase is marked by a loss of cohesin along the chromatid arms and separation of the arms.

2. B. Histone acetylation and active transcription of that gene go hand in hand. Euchromatin is associated with active gene transcription and has more histone acetylation. Heterochromatin, with less gene activ-ity, has less histone acetylation. The centromere is composed of α-satellite DNA, a form of repetitive transcriptionally inactive DNA. Kinetochores and mitotic spindles are made of proteins, not DNA.

3. C. Condensins are a hallmark of metaphase and are activated by M-cyclin–dependent kinase. The mitotic spindle and the associated microtubules also form, but initially the existing cytoplasmic microtubules must be degraded.

4. A. Paclitaxel interferes with normal mitosis. To be affected by an antimitotic drug, a cell must either be capable of cell division or undergo relatively rapid cell division. Bone marrow stem cells are engaged in constant cell division to replenish the cells which originate from the bone marrow (red blood cells, white blood cells, platelets). Any other cell that is actively dividing—hair follicles, gastrointestinal epithelium, sperm, or the out-of-control cancer cell—is likely to be affected by an antimitotic drug. Central nervous system neurons in the postembryonic period are no longer dividing. Mature red blood cells and the outer layer of skin epithelial cells have lost their nuclei and are no longer capable of mitosis.

5. B. Bloom syndrome. Gout is a defect of uric acid metabolism. Down syndrome is caused by an extra chromosome 21. Scleroderma is an autoimmune disorder in which an individual may form antibodies against the centromere–kinetochore apparatus.

CHAPTER 3

1. B. Because the couple is not pregnant, choices A and C are not appropriate. Neurons (E) do not actively divide and are not suitable for cytogenetic analysis.

Gonadal tissue (D) is more difficult to obtain, particularly in women, and would be less suitable than a blood sample.

2. C. Light-banded regions of chromosomes are GC-rich and more heavily transcribed (euchromatin). Centromeres and heterochromatin are dark banded. The nucleolar organizing regions are the p arms of acrocentric chromosomes with repetitive copies of genes encoding rRNA.

3. A. No acrocentric chromosomes are involved; therefore, any type of Robertsonian translocation is incorrect. Paracentric inversions are within a single chromosome. The normal phenotype implies that the translocation is balanced rather than unbalanced.

B. The clinical picture of a girl with short stature and learning disability is consistent with Turner syndrome (45,X). A child with Down syndrome has more severe developmental disability, more consistent with mental retardation. A girl with triple X syndrome has tall stature.

4. B. The intrauterine growth retardation, heart defect, and unusual clenched hands are clinical features typical of trisomy 18, an aneuploid condition caused by maternal meiotic nondisjunction.

5. C. Chorionic villus sampling can be performed earlier in gestation than other prenatal diagnostic methods. It samples extraembryonic cells that must be cultured longer than blood cells. In addition, it is not capable of detecting fetal proteins, which may be present in amniotic fluid.

CHAPTER 4

1. B. Klinefelter males who carry an abnormal X gene are affected by it in the same way as 46,XX females: random X inactivation determines which cells and tissues express the abnormal gene. The effect on the phenotype is determined by the number of cells and specific cells expressing the abnormal gene.

2. E. PCR is the only response that amplifies DNA.

3. D. Microarray analysis is the only response that permits evaluation of gene expression.

4. A. A DNA polymorphism should have minimal impact on gene function and is frequently silent (no change in amino acid). A Western blot should detect normal amounts of protein. The polymorphism is in an exon, so measure of intronic segments is not helpful. Both copies of *COL2A1* should be present as detected by FISH.

5. E. α-Satellite and β-satellite DNA is present in areas of heterochromatin, usually at or near the centromere. Microsatellite DNA is interspersed throughout the genome and consists of repeats of 1 to 4 nucleotides.

CHAPTER 5

1. E. Sunburn is caused by ultraviolet light associated with covalent bonding of adjacent thymidine bases. Breaks in DNA strands are caused by ionizing radiation, such as γ-radiation.

2. B. Defects in DNA repair mechanisms allow accumulation of somatic mutations in DNA. Somatic mutations occurring within genes responsible for cellular growth and control ultimately lead to uncontrolled cell growth or cancer. Some DNA repair defects cause dominant disorders, such as hereditary breast/ovarian cancer syndrome or hereditary nonpolyposis colorectal cancer. These dominant disorders are found in adults with normal mental and physical development.

3. B. Gain-of-function mutations are always missense mutations, and they occur in highly specific regions of a gene, limiting the variability of location. In contrast, dominant negative mutations have more variation within the same gene. Haploinsufficiency and null alleles are associated with reductions in protein production. Polymorphism does not produce a disease phenotype.

4. A. The association of a common disease phenotype, achondroplasia, with a single missense mutation strongly supports a gain-of-function mutation as the cause. Loss-of-function mutations (B, C, and D) are more varied in form. Recessive effects (E) are usually caused by loss-of-function mutations.

CHAPTER 6

1. D. Refer to Figure 6.6 for discussion. III-3 is the unaffected sister of a female with an autosomal recessive disorder. Her parents must both be heterozygotes. Since she is unaffected, she cannot have an aa genotype. She has three other options: AA, Aa, or aA. She has a two in three chance of being a heterozygote. If only one of her parents were a carrier, she would have a 50% chance of also being a carrier, but then it would not be possible for her to have an affected sister. The other choices are fillers.

2. B. The question asks which individuals must be heterozygotes, therefore, which are obligate heterozygotes. The answers are explained fully in the answer section for Figure 6.9, discussed after the next question.

3. C. Amniocentesis is not appropriate, because amniocytes do not express the biochemical abnormality. Cordocentesis at 28 weeks is too late to allow pregnancy termination in the event of an affected child. Preimplantation genetic diagnosis is not possible, because no mutation was detected and biochemical analysis cannot be done on single cells. Ultrasonography does not detect the features of Menkes syndrome. The only remaining answer is chorionic villus sampling. Chorionic villus sampling will permit biochemical analysis in the fetal chorionic cells, which have a different cellular origin from that of amniocytes and which express the defect in copper metabolism.

Answers to questions for Figure 6.9:

- The inheritance pattern may be autosomal dominant, because of the females and male affected. Individual III-3 is a problem. Inheritance seems unlikely to be autosomal recessive because of the number of affected generations. X-linked inheritance also seems unlikely because an affected female passed the disease through an unaffected male to another affected female.
  - III-3 in an autosomal dominant setting would have to carry the mutated allele to pass it to his daughter. He just does not have any symptoms from his allele. This does not seem possible using mendelian genetic theories.
  - Three affected generations may occur if the heterozygote frequency in the population is higher than is typically seen in autosomal recessive disorders.
  - X is theoretically possible, because the same X could be transmitted from II-5 to III-3 to IV-2. It is unlikely, since this pattern does not fit either X-linked recessive or X-linked dominant phenotypic patterns. It cannot be on the Y because of the female-to-male transmission pattern from II-5 to III-3.
  - It is not possible to determine definitively the inheritance pattern from the available information.
- The presence of congenital symptoms in all affected individuals permits the deduction that III-3 really is not likely to have the disease.
  - If III-3 is truly unaffected, the inheritance pattern is not likely to be dominant, either.
- The use of bioinformatics is a critical tool in the diagnosis of rare genetic disorders. It is not possible for any single practitioner to know every rare and obscure disorder.
  - Any parent of an affected child should be considered a heterozygote unless molecular testing diagnoses an unusual situation, such as false parenthood or uniparental disomy. Obligate heterozygotes are I-3, I-4, II-4, III-3, and III-4.
  - Either I-1 or I-2 is a heterozygote. It is not possible to determine which one from the available information. As the couple did not have any affected children, it is unlikely that they are both heterozygotes. Except for the obligate heterozygotes, all unaffected individuals (II-1, II-2, II-3, II-6, IV-1) are possible heterozygotes.
  - Factors which could contribute to the high number of obligate heterozygotes include a closed population with a high proportion of consanguinity or founder effect or a disorder that has a high heterozygote frequency.

There is no way of determining from the available information the frequency of heterozygotes in the general population.

CHAPTER 7

1. E. While oxidative phosphorylation reactions occur primarily in the mitochondria, other metabolic processes occur also. Age of onset alone does not refute mitochondrial inheritance, since the mother may have a lower frequency of abnormal mitochondria in her somatic cells than in her germ cells. Either males or females may have a mitochondrially inherited disorder, but only females can transmit it to the next generation. If the disorder was mitochondrially inherited, all offspring of the mother should have symptoms.

2. B. An isolated population is likely to be a founder population with a high gene and carrier frequency for some autosomal or X-linked recessive disorders.

3. E. Neurofibromatosis is the prototype disorder for variable expressivity. The symptoms described in different family members indicate the range of features found in this family.

4. C. The student does not need to remember that achondroplasia was described in the text as an autosomal dominant disorder. The statement that it is caused by a mutation in one copy of the gene signifies a dominant disorder. A de novo or new mutation is the only option among those listed, since the parents do not have the disorder.

5. D. Uniparental disomy is defined as receipt of both copies of a chromosome from the same parent. Uniparental disomy was not specifically mentioned in Chapter 7, but the student should be able to synthesize and recall the information from earlier chapters.

CHAPTER 8

1. B. The pedigree is consistent with hereditary breast/ovarian cancer syndrome, with two occurrences of premenopausal breast cancer and one ovarian cancer. The syndrome is caused by a mutation in either *BRCA1* or *BRCA2*. The other genes in the other choices are for the following inherited cancer susceptibility syndromes:
  i.   Chronic myeloid leukemia
  ii. Hereditary nonpolyposis colorectal cancer
  iii. Multiple endocrine neoplasia type 2 and hereditary papillary renal carcinoma
  iv. Li-Fraumeni syndrome and Cowden syndrome

2. D. Individual II-3 is an obligate carrier of the genetic mutation, since he is the connection between II-5 and III-1. He is nonpenetrant for hereditary breast/ovarian cancer syndrome because of his gender. III-1 was not spared from the hereditary disorder, as would be expected in (A). Hereditary breast/ovarian cancer syndrome is not involved in imprinting (C). The genetic mutation was transmitted to II-3 so the nonpenetrance in I-2 is not responsible (E).

3. D. Individual III-2 is concerned because she has both a maternal and a paternal history of premenopausal-onset breast cancer. As in all susceptibility testing, it is important to begin testing with an affected individual. This eliminates choices A, B, and E. Individuals II-6 and III-1 have both had cancer, but III-1 (D) is the best option because she is a first-degree relative to III-2 and had an earlier onset of cancer. In addition, II-6 is separated from III-2 by three nonpenetrant individuals and could represent a phenocopy.

4. C. Ashkenazi Jews have a 2 to 3% risk of carrying a deleterious *BRCA1* or *BRCA2* founder mutation. African Americans (A) have a 50% likelihood of a variant of uncertain significance but a much smaller risk of deleterious mutations than do Jews. Choices B, D, and E are not associated with any increased risk.

CHAPTER 9

1. B. The twins are monozygotic, because they are of the same sex and have an identical tandem repeat pattern in their DNA.

With monozygotic twins, there should be no difference in the existence of single-gene disorders, eliminating choices A, C, and E. Monozygotic twins may differ in the phenotypic expression of complex disorders, because they may be exposed to different intrauterine microenvironments. Depending on the timing of separation of the zygote, the twins could have separate placentas and amniotic sacs, a single placenta and separate amniotic sacs, or a single placenta and sac. Microenvironments may differ even with a single sac and placenta because of differences in umbilical cord blood supply. Questionable paternity (choice D) would affect both monozygotic twins, not just one.

2. **E.** The low concordance level between monozygotic twins diminishes the likelihood of any significant genetic contribution to the disorder. The similar concordance levels between monozygotic and dizygotic twins and the discrepancy with concordance in siblings increase the likelihood of a prenatal environmental component.

3. **B.** The 100% concordance between monozygotic twins implies mendelian inheritance. A 25% concordance with dizygotic twins and siblings is consistent with autosomal recessive inheritance.

4. **B.** The unborn child is a first-degree relative of the affected father. Regardless of the fact that the existing children are normal, the risk of cleft lip or palate in future siblings is 3 to 4%. However, if any of the siblings had been affected, the risk of any future child being affected would be higher because the presence of a background combination of genetic and environmental factors has been demonstrated.

5. **E.** The man discovers that he has a significant genetic risk for schizophrenia based on the diagnosis in his identical twin and a sibling. Schizophrenia also has a strong environmental effect, particularly if an affected parent is involved. The upper end of the range for identical twins (79%) would be expected in monozygotic twins who also shared the same childhood environment. The lower end (44%) would be more ex-

pected for twins reared apart, as in this case. However, the additional affected sibling implies that additional genetic factors may be present.

CHAPTER 10

1. **D.** The tongue failed to descend into the oropharynx, which served as a mechanical factor preventing the closure of the palatal shelves. Box 10.1 defines sequence as resulting from a mechanical factor leading to multiple secondary effects.

2. **C.** The ventricular septum failed to form because of intrinsically abnormal development (malformation). It never existed in the first place (necessary feature of either a disruption or a deformation). No mechanical factor contributed (needed for sequence).

3. **C.** The existence of testes implies that a functional *SRY* gene is present or gonadal differentiation would not have occurred. No müllerian structures are present; therefore, antimüllerian hormone was present. An elevated testosterone level implies blockage after testosterone synthesis, but total lack of the androgen receptor should result in female external genitalia with blind vaginal pouch rather than ambiguous genitalia. A deficiency of 5α-reductase type 2 is consistent with the phenotype described.

CHAPTER 11

1. **E.** The CYP3A enzyme family is involved in oxidative metabolism rather than acetylation, hydroxylation, or interaction with surface receptors. If it is induced, function of other hepatic metabolic processes also tends to be increased.

2. **A.** Ultrarapid metabolizers have multiple copies of the *CYP2D6* gene (amplification). Anticipation, gain-of-function mutations, and frameshift mutations are not involved in amplification. Induction of hepatic enzymes may produce an increase in activity within a single individual but does not affect entire populations.

CHAPTER 12

1. A. Of the vectors listed, only adeno-associated virus, a type of parvovirus, is known to insert its gene into the host genome. Adenovirus, liposomes, and naked DNA transfer do not. Retroviruses are also capable of insertion.

2. E. Adeno-associated virus, a type of parvovirus, inserts into the genome preferentially at 19q13.3 rather than near the promoter of any actively expressing gene. Adenovirus and naked DNA transfer do not insert into the genome. Retrovirus is known to insert near the promoter.

Glossary

actin: Protein that along with myosin is the main component of muscle. Molecules of actin come together (polymerize) to form long regularly-aligned filaments.

adeno-associated viral vector (AAV): Non-pathogenic human parvoviruses capable of infecting both dividing and nondividing cells; can integrate into a specific point of the host genome (19q13-qter).

adenoviral vector: DNA derived from adenoviruses and used for studies of gene transfer; usually deleted for one or more early viral genes (most commonly E1and E3 deleted). Because of these deletions, require specialized cell lines (so-called producer cells) in which to propagate.

aflatoxin: Potent hepatotoxic and hepatocarcinogenic mycotoxin produced by the aspergillus flavus group of fungi; found as a contaminant in peanuts, cottonseed meal, corn, and other grains.

alkylating agent: Substance containing an alkyl group which can be inserted into an organic compound; can act on DNA and interfere with replication, making it useful for destroying rapidly dividing cells, such as cancer cells.

allelic heterogeneity: Single disorder, trait, or pattern of traits caused by different mutations within a gene.

alternative splicing: Production of two or more distinct mRNAs from an RNA transcript through the choice of different exons and differences in splicing.

amniocentesis: Prenatal diagnosis method using cells in the amniotic fluid to determine the number and kind of chromosomes of the fetus and, when indicated, perform biochemical studies.

anaphase: Stage of meiosis or mitosis when chromosomes move toward opposite ends of the nuclear spindle.

anticipation: Phenomenon in which a genetic condition appears to become more severe and/or appear at an earlier age with subsequent generations.

association: Statistical relationship between two or more events, characteristics, or other variables.

autosome: Any chromosome that is not one of the sex chromosomes. The diploid human genome consists of 46 chromosomes, 22 pairs of autosomes, and one pair of sex chromosomes (the X and Y chromosomes).

balanced reciprocal translocation: Chromosome alteration in which a whole chromosome or segment of a chromosome becomes attached to or interchanged with another whole chromosome or segment, the resulting hybrid segregating together at meiosis; balanced translocations (in which there is no net loss or gain of chromosome material) are usually not associated with phenotypic abnormalities, although gene disruptions at the breakpoints of the translocation can in some cases cause adverse effects, including some known genetic disorders.

Barr body: The condensed single X-chromosome seen in the nuclei of somatic cells of individuals with more than one X chromosome.

base excision repair: An altered base is removed by a DNA glycosylase enzyme, followed by excision of the resulting sugar phosphate. The small gap left in the DNA helix is filled in by the sequential action of DNA polymerase and DNA ligase.

carcinogenesis: Process by which normal cells are transformed into cancer cells.

carcinoma: Any malignant tumor derived from epithelial tissue.

cell cycle: Sequence of events a cell goes through during replication as seen from mitotic event to mitotic event.

centromere: Constricted portion of the metaphase chromosome at which the chromatids are joined and by which the chromosome is attached to the spindle during cell division.

centrosome: Primary microtubule-organizing center of animal cells; divides prior to cell division. Each daughter centrosome acts as one pole of the spindle apparatus and contains a pair of centrioles.

chiasma (plural, chiasmata): Reciprocal recombination event in meiosis, observable in the later stage of meiotic prophase. Chiasmata hold homologous chromosomes together prior to anaphase of the first meiotic division.

chorionic villus sampling: An invasive prenatal diagnostic procedure involving removal of villi from the human chorion to obtain chromosomes and cell products for diagnosis of disorders in the human embryo.

chromatid: One of the two daughter strands of a duplicated chromosome.

chromatin: The nuclear material that makes up chromosomes, consisting of DNA and protein.

chromosome painting: A technique for visualizing chromosome abnormalities using fluorescence-labeled DNA probes hybridized to chromosomal DNA. A variety of fluorescent labels may be attached to the probes. Upon hybridization, a multicolored, or painted, effect is produced with a unique color at each site of hybridization.

clinical heterogeneity: Differences in clinical presentation of the same disorder.

clone: Organism derived from a founding individual by asexual means that is genetically identical to the founding individual.

cloning: Using specialized DNA technology to produce multiple exact copies of a single gene or other segment of DNA to obtain enough material for further study.

cohesin: Protein that acts as glue joining two sister chromatids along their lengths.

comparative genomic hybridization: Molecular cytogenetic technique used for analysis of DNA content in malignant tumor cells. DNA from tumor tissue and from normal control tissue (reference) is labeled with different colors and mixed. The mix is hybridized to normal metaphase chromosomes. The fluorescence color ratio along the chromosomes is used to evaluate regions of DNA gain or loss in the tumor sample.

concordance: Presence of a given trait in both members of a pair of twins.

condensin: Protein complex that organizes chromosomes into their highly compact mitotic structure.

confined placental mosaicism: Tissue-specific mosaicism affecting the placenta only.

consanguinity: Degree of relationship between persons who descend from a common ancestor.

cordocentesis: Procedure to sample umbilical cord blood during pregnancy.

CpG island: DNA region characterized by methylated cytosine residues in the sequence CpG.

crossing over: Genetic recombination through transfer of genetic material between two homologous DNA regions; recombination.

cyclin: protein active in regulating the cell cycle.

cyclin-dependent kinase: protein kinase involved in regulation of the cell cycle, activated by association with a cyclin forming a cyclin-dependent kinase complex.

cytokinesis: Division of the cytoplasm of a cell into two daughter cells.

cytosine deamination: Removal of the amino group from a cytosine residue. Spontaneous deamination is the hydrolysis reaction of cytosine into uracil. Spontaneous deamination of 5-methylcytosine results in thymine. In DNA, this reaction cannot be corrected because the repair mechanisms do not recognize thymine (as opposed to uracil) as erroneous. This flaw in the repair mechanism contributes to the rarity of CpG sites in the eukaryotic genome.

denaturing high-performance liquid chromatography: Method for screening DNA samples for single nucleotide polymorphisms and inherited mutations.

de novo mutation: Alteration in a gene that is present for the first time in one family member as a result of a mutation in a germ cell (egg or sperm) of one of the parents or in the fertilized egg itself.

diploid: Having twice the chromosome number normally found in a gamete.

differentiation: Process in embryonic development during which unspecialized cells or tissues become specialized for particular functions.

directive counseling: Counseling which tells and advises.

dizygotic twins: Twins developed from two separate fertilized eggs; fraternal twins.

dominant: Allele that is almost always expressed, even if only one copy is present.

dominant negative: Mutation whose gene product adversely affects the normal, wild-type gene product within the same cell, usually by dimerizing with it. In cases of polymeric molecules, dominant negative mutations are often more deleterious than mutations causing the production of no gene product (null mutations or null alleles).

duplication: Extra copy of a DNA segment in the genome.

dysmorphology: Clinical study of malformation syndromes.

epigenetics: Heritable changes in gene function that occur without a change in the sequence of nuclear DNA.

euchromatin: Part of the genome characterized by relatively high gene density and relative absence of highly repetitive sequences.

exon: Protein-coding DNA sequence of a gene.

familial: Tending to occur in more members of a family than expected by chance alone.

first-degree relative: Any relative who is one meiosis away from a particular individual in a family (i.e., parent, sibling, offspring).

fluorescence in situ hybridization (FISH): Cytogenetic technique used to identify the presence of specific chromosomes or chromosomal regions through hybridization of fluorescence-labeled DNA probes to denatured chromosomal DNA. Examination under fluorescent lighting detects the presence (hybridized fluorescent signal) or absence (no hybridized fluorescent signal) of the chromosome material.

founder effect: Lack of genetic diversity occurring when a small population establishes itself in isolation.

frameshift mutation: Addition or deletion of a nucleotide to a DNA sequence, causing out-of-phase translation.

G-banding: Technique for producing banding patterns in eukaryotic chromosomes. Bands are produced by staining with Giemsa stain after pretreating chromosomes with trypsin. Each homologous chromosome pair has a unique pattern of G-bands, enabling recognition of particular chromosomes.

gain-of-function mutation: Mutation that creates a new or enhanced function for a gene, usually capable of expression in the heterozygous state (dominant).

gene therapy: Replacement of an individual's faulty genetic material with normal genetic material to treat or cure a disease or abnormal medical condition.

germ cells: Sperm and egg cells and their precursors. Germ cells are haploid, having only one set of chromosomes (23 in humans), while all other human cells have two copies (46).

germline mosaicism (gonadal mosaicism): Two or more genetic or cytogenetic cell lines confined to the germ cells; formerly called gonadal mosaicism.

haploid: Having only a single set of chromosomes (half of the full set of genetic material); present in the egg and sperm cells of animals and in the egg and pollen cells of plants. Human beings have 23 chromosomes in their reproductive cells.

haploinsufficiency: Situation in which an individual who is heterozygous for a certain gene mutation is clinically affected because a single copy of the normal gene is incapable of providing sufficient protein production to ensure normal function.

heterochromatin: The part of the genome characterized by relatively low gene density and highly repetitive sequences. Heterochromatin is more highly condensed than euchromatin.

heteroduplex: DNA double helix formed by annealing single strands from different sources; if there is a sequence difference between the strands, the heteroduplex may show single strand loops or bubbles (unpaired regions).

heteroplasmy: Mixture of mitochondria within a single cell, some containing mutant DNA and some containing normal DNA.

homogeneously staining regions: Amplification of DNA sequences in tumor cells which can appear as extra or expanded areas of the chromosomes which stain evenly.

homolog: 1. One member of a chromosome pair. **2.** Gene similar in structure and evolutionary origin to a gene in another species.

immunohistochemistry: Use of antibodies to proteins (antigens) as histological tools for identifying patterns of antigen distribution within a tissue or an organism. An antibody that binds to a specific protein is tagged with a fluorescent chemical or an enzyme that can convert a substrate to a visible dye. The tagged antibody is incubated with the tissue, and after unbound antibody is washed away, the bound antibody distribution is revealed by fluorescence microscopy or incubation with a chromogenic substrate. It is assumed that antibody distribution reflects antigen distribution.

imprinting: Epigenetic modification of genes that identifies a given gene as having been inherited from the maternal or paternal parent. In mammals, some genes are expressed primarily from the maternally inherited or paternally inherited alleles as a consequence of imprinting.

inbreeding: Mating among related individuals which reduces genetic diversity and may lead to expression of deleterious recessive characteristics and reduction of fitness in the offspring.

induction: Synthesis of a gene product or products in response to the action of a chemical or environmental agent.

informed consent: Consent to a medical procedure by a patient who possesses and understands all of the information necessary to make a reasoned decision. Clinicians have an obligation to allow patients to be active participants in decision making regarding their care or participation in research. Informed consent, rooted in the concept of autonomous choice, or the right of self-determination, includes five elements: disclosure of information to the patient, comprehension by the patient of the information being disclosed, voluntariness of the patient in making the choice, competence of the patient to make a decision, and consent by the patient.

insertion: Type of mutation in which one or more nucleotides is inserted into a DNA sequence that can alter the reading frame and thus the amino acid sequence of the encoded protein.

interphase: Stage of a cell not undergoing mitosis or meiosis. Interphase includes G1, S, and G2 phases of the cell division cycle.

interstitial deletion: Deletion of a section of genetic material within a chromosome, not involving the telomere.

intron: Noncoding DNA sequence within a gene that is initially transcribed into messenger RNA but is later spliced out.

inversion: Type of mutation in which a length of DNA is broken in two positions and repaired in such a way that the segment is in reverse order.

karyotype: Photomicrograph of an individual's chromosomes arranged in a standard format showing the number, size, and shape of each chromosome type; used in low-resolution physical mapping to correlate gross chromosomal abnormalities with the characteristics of specific diseases.

kinetochore: Structure formed adjacent to the centromere of a condensed chromosome that allows the chromosome to attach to microtubules of the meiotic or mitotic spindle.

linkage: Use of several DNA sequence polymorphisms (normal variants) that are near or within a gene of interest to track within a family the inheritance of a disease-causing mutation in that gene; indirect DNA analysis.

liposomes: Artificial single or multilaminar vesicles (made from lecithins or other lipids) used to deliver a variety of biological molecules or molecular complexes to cells, for example, drug delivery and gene transfer.

locus heterogeneity: Single disorder, trait, or pattern of traits caused by mutations in genes at different chromosomal loci.

loss-of-function mutation: Mutation in an allele that results in the loss of the function for which it normally encodes. The function may be reduced or entirely lost (null mutation or null allele).

metaphase: Stage in mitosis or meiosis during which the chromosomes are aligned along the equatorial plane of the cell.

microarray: Tool used to sift through and analyze the information in a genome; consists of nucleic acid probes chemically attached to a substrate, which can be a microchip, a glass slide, or a microsphere bead.

microsatellite DNA: Repetitive segments of DNA 2 to 5 nucleotides in length (dinucleotide-trinucleotide-tetranucleotide repeats), scattered throughout the genome, often used as markers for linkage analysis because of high variability in repeat number between individuals. These regions are inherently unstable and susceptible to mutations.

microtubule: Cytoskeletal element of eukaryotic cells; a long, generally straight, hollow tube with an external diameter of 24 nm, consisting of polymerized monomers of tubulin. Microtubules make up the bulk of the spindle.

minisatellite DNA: Repeated segments of the same sequence, each segment varying between 14 and 100 base pairs, useful as linkage markers because of their highly polymorphic nature and the fact that they are usually situated near genes. Minisatellites are inherently unstable, susceptible to mutation at a higher rate than other sequences of DNA.

mismatch repair: DNA proofreading system controlled by certain genes that identifies, excises, and corrects errors in pairing of bases during DNA replication.

missense mutation: Single–base pair substitution that results in translation of a different amino acid at that position.

mitotic spindle: Fusiform figure characteristic of a dividing cell, consisting of microtubules, some of which become attached to each chromosome at its centromere and provide the mechanism for chromosomal movement.

modifier gene: Gene that alters the effect produced by another gene.

monozygotic twins: Twins who originate from one egg and one sperm; identical twins.

morphogen: Soluble molecules that can diffuse and carry signals to control cell differentiation decisions in a concentration-dependent fashion; typically act by binding to specific protein receptors.

morphogenesis: Aspect of developmental biology concerned with the shapes of tissues, organs, and entire organisms; positions of the various specialized cell types; and processes that control the organized spatial distribution of cells.

multigenic trait: Hereditary characteristic that is specified by several genes.

multipoint linkage: Use of multiple DNA single-nucleotide polymorphisms in a region to narrow the genomic location of a gene of interest.

multipotent: Describing a cell or tissue able to form several kinds of cells or tissues but committed to producing cells with a particular function; e.g., blood stem cells are multipotent: they can produce red blood cells, white blood cells, and platelets.

mutation: Any alteration in a gene from its natural state; may be disease causing or a benign, normal variant.

myosin: Contractile protein that interacts with actin to bring about contraction of muscle or cell movement. Myosin is present in the myofibrils of the muscles.

nondirective counseling: Counseling which reflects what is said and felt; assists with decision making without suggesting a particular decision.

nondisjunction: Failure of homologous chromosomes or chromatids to segregate during mitosis or meiosis with the result that one daughter cell has both of a pair of parental chromosomes or chromatids and the other has none.

nonsense mutation: Single–base pair substitution that prematurely codes for a stop in amino acid translation (stop codon).

nucleosome: Unit of DNA and histones. Multiple units make up chromatin found in the nucleus of eukaryotes.

null allele: Allele whose effect is either absence of normal gene product at the molecular level or absence of normal function at the phenotypic level.

oncogene: Gene having the potential to cause a normal cell to become cancerous.

paracentric inversion: Inversion in which the breakpoints are confined to one arm of a chromosome; the inverted segment does not span the centromere.

pedigree: Diagram of the genetic relationships and medical history of a family using standardized symbols and terminology.

penetrance: Proportion of individuals with a mutation causing a particular disorder who exhibit clinical symptoms of that disorder; a condition (most commonly inherited in an autosomal dominant manner) is said to have complete penetrance if clinical symptoms are present in all individuals who have the disease-causing mutation and to have reduced or incomplete penetrance if clinical symptoms are not always present in individuals who have the disease-causing mutation.

pericentric inversion: Inversion in which the breakpoints occur on both arms of a chromosome. The inverted segment spans the centromere.

pharmacogenetics: Study of the way drugs interact with genetic makeup; genetic response to a drug.

pharmacogenomics: Analysis of the effect of genetic variation (polymorphisms) on drug response; has the potential to help clinicians administer tailored treatment; often refers specifically to tests that predict drug response; however, *pharmacogenetics* and *pharmacogenomics* are often used interchangeably.

phenocopy: Trait not caused by inheritance of a gene but appearing to be identical to a genetic trait.

pluripotent: Able to give rise to many but not all types of cells.

polygenic trait: Trait resulting from the combined action of alleles of more than one gene (e.g., heart disease, diabetes, some cancers). Although such disorders are inherited, they depend on the simultaneous presence of several alleles; thus the hereditary patterns usually are more complex than those of single-gene disorders.

polymerase chain reaction: Procedure that produces multiple copies of a short segment of DNA through cycles of (*a*) denaturation (heat-induced separation of double-stranded DNA into single strands); (*b*) annealing (binding of specific primers on either end of the target segment); and (*c*) elongation (extension of the primer sequences over the target segment with DNA polymerase). The amplified product, doubled each cycle for 30 or more cycles, can be subjected to further testing.

polymorphism: Natural variations in a gene, DNA sequence, or chromosome that have no adverse effects on the individual and occur with fairly high frequency in the general population.

prometaphase: Stage between the prophase and metaphase of mitosis or meiosis; characterized by disappearance of the nuclear membrane and formation of the spindle.

prophase: First stage of mitosis. The individual chromosomes of the cell become clearly visible within the nucleus with a light microscope as they condense from long, thin, wispy structures to thick structures, and they appear as a tangled jumble of paired identical chromatids. By late prophase, the nuclear membrane disappears and all of the chromosomes are fully condensed.

proto-oncogene: Gene that normally directs cell growth but if altered (becoming an oncogene) can promote or allow the uncontrolled growth of cancer. Alterations can be inherited or caused by an environmental exposure to carcinogens.

pseudogene: Copy of a gene that usually lacks introns and other essential DNA sequences necessary for function. Pseudogenes, though genetically similar to the original functional gene, are not expressed and often contain numerous mutations.

reactive oxygen species: Reactive intermediate oxygen species including both radicals and nonradicals. These substances are constantly formed in the human body, have been shown to kill bacteria and inactivate proteins, and have been implicated in a number of diseases, such as cancer development.

recessive: Gene that is phenotypically manifest in the homozygous state but masked in the presence of a dominant allele.

recombination: Exchange of a segment of DNA between two homologous chromosomes during meiosis leading to a novel combination of genetic material in the offspring; crossing over.

recombination repair: Repair of a DNA lesion through a process similar to recombination that uses recombination enzymes.

relative risk: Quantitative measure used to describe the increase or decrease in risk associated with a specific risk factor. A relative risk is the ratio of two absolute risks: the numerator is the absolute risk among those with the risk factor, and the denominator is the absolute risk among those without the risk factor.

reproductive cloning: Making a full living copy of an organism; requires a surrogate mother.

retroviral vector: Artificial DNA construct derived from a retrovirus, used to insert sequences into an organism's chromosomes.

robertsonian translocation: Joining of two acrocentric chromosomes at the centromeres with loss of their short arms to form a single abnormal chromosome; acrocentric chromosomes are the Y chromosome and chromosomes 13, 14, 15, 21, and 22.

sarcoma: Cancer of the bone, cartilage, fat, muscle, blood vessels, or other connective or supportive tissue.

satellite DNA: Fraction of a eukaryotic organism's DNA that differs in density from most of its DNA as determined by centrifugation, that consists of short repetitive nucleotide sequences, that does not undergo transcription, and that is often found in centromeric regions.

second-degree relative: Any relative who is two meioses away from a particular individual in a pedigree; a relative with whom one quarter of an individual's genes is shared (i.e., grandparent, grandchild, uncle, aunt, nephew, niece, half-sibling).

silent mutation: Mutation that does not change the amino acid sequence or product of the gene.

single nucleotide polymorphism: DNA sequence variations that occur when a single nucleotide (A, T, C, or G) in the genome sequence is altered.

sister chromatid exchange: Reciprocal exchange of DNA between the two DNA molecules of a replicating chromosome.

somatic cell: Any cell of a multicellular organism that does not participate in the production of reproductive or germ line cells. Somatic cells differentiate to specialized cells with a limited potential to divide.

somatic cell gene therapy: Incorporation of new genetic material into cells for therapeutic purposes. The new genetic material cannot be passed to offspring.

somatic mosaicism: Two or more genetic or cytogenetic cell lines within the cells of the body (may or may not include the germline cells).

spectral karyotype: Visualization of all of an organism's chromosomes together, each labeled with a different color, useful for identifying chromosome abnormalities.

spliceosome: Ribonucleoprotein complex that is the site in the cell nucleus where introns are excised from precursor messenger RNA and exons are joined together to form functional messenger RNA.

stem cell: Relatively undifferentiated cells of the same lineage that retain the ability to divide and cycle throughout postnatal life to provide cells that can become specialized and take the place of those that die or are lost.

synaptonemal complex: Structure that holds paired chromosomes together during prophase I of meiosis and that promotes genetic recombination.

tandem repeats: Two identical DNA sequences arranged one behind the other in varying numbers. These regions are hypervariable because of unequal crossing over or slippage during replication.

telomerase: Enzyme complex that maintains chromosome ends; referred to as a cellular immortalizing enzyme. Telomerase is composed of both RNA and proteins. Its internal RNA component is complementary to the telomeric single-stranded overhang, multiple repeats of the sequence TTAGGG. Telomerase uses its internal RNA as a template for synthesis of telomeric DNA directly onto the ends of chromosomes. Telomerase is present in most fetal tissues, normal adult male germ cells, inflammatory cells, proliferative cells of renewal tissues, and most tumor cells.

telomere: Segment at the end of each chromosome arm consisting of a series of repeated DNA sequences, believed to be a few hundred base pairs long, that regulate chromosomal replication at each cell division. Some of the telomere is lost each time a cell divides, and eventually, when the telomere is gone, the cell dies.

telophase: Terminal stage of mitosis or meiosis in which chromosomes uncoil, the spindle breaks down, and cytokinesis usually occurs.

therapeutic cloning: Nuclear transplantation of a patient's own cells to make an oocyte from which immune-compatible cells (especially stem cells) can be derived for transplant.

third-degree relative: Any relative who is three meioses away from a particular individual in a pedigree; a relative with whom one-eighth of an individual's genes is shared (i.e., great grandparent, great grandchild, first cousin).

thymidine dimer: Pair of abnormally chemically bonded adjacent thymine bases in

DNA, resulting from damage by ultraviolet irradiation.

totipotent: Having unlimited capability. Totipotent cells have the capacity to specialize into extraembryonic membranes and tissues, the embryo, and all postembryonic tissues and organs.

transcription factor: Any of various proteins that bind to DNA and play a role in the regulation of gene expression by promoting transcription.

triplet repeat: Sequences of three nucleotides repeated in tandem on the same chromosome a number of times. A normal polymorphic variation in repeat number with no clinical significance commonly occurs between individuals; however, repeat numbers over a certain threshold can in some cases lead to adverse effects on the function of the gene, resulting in genetic disease.

triploidy: Three haploid sets of chromosomes in a single cell (in humans, a total of 69 chromosomes per cell).

tubulin: Protein subunit of microtubules.

tumor suppressor gene: Gene that normally restrains cell growth; cells grow uncontrolled when it is missing or inactivated by mutation.

ubiquitin: Protein that is covalently attached to lysines of other proteins, tagging them for proteolysis within proteasomes.

ultraviolet radiation: Electromagnetic radiation with wavelengths ranging from 1 to 300 nm. Can be divided into three types: UVA (responsible for tanning the skin and some types of skin cancers), UVB (responsible for sunburn and skin cancers), and UVC (potentially lethal radiation, but does not reach the earth's surface because of protection from the ozone layer).

unbalanced translocation: Chromosome alteration in which a whole chromosome or a segment of one becomes attached to or interchanged with another whole chromosome or segment, the resulting hybrid segregating together at meiosis; unbalanced translocations (in which there is loss or gain of chromosome material) nearly always yield an abnormal phenotype.

unequal crossing over: Mispairing and exchange of DNA between genetically similar nonhomologous chromosome regions that results in duplication or deletion of DNA in each daughter cell.

uniparental disomy (UPD): Situation in which both members of a chromosome pair or segments of a chromosome pair are inherited from one parent and neither is inherited from the other parent. Uniparental disomy can result in an abnormal phenotype in some cases.

unipotent: Capable of developing into only one type of cell or tissue.

variable expression: Variation in clinical features (type and severity) of a genetic disorder between individuals with the same gene alteration, even within the same family.

X chromosome inactivation: In females, the phenomenon by which one X chromosome (either maternally or paternally derived) is randomly inactivated in early embryonic cells, with fixed inactivation in all descendant cells; first described by the geneticist Mary Lyon; lyonization.

Table of Genes Referenced

GENE SYMBOL	CHAPTERS	OMIM[a] NUMBER	NAME	LOCATION	ALTERNATIVE TITLES AND SYMBOLS
ABCB1	11	171050	ATP-binding cassette, subfamily B, member 1	7q21.1	P-glycoprotein 1: PGY1; multidrug resistance 1: MDR1; GP170; doxorubicin resistance
ABL	8	189980	Abelson murine leukemia viral oncogene homolog 1	9q34.1	Transformation gene: oncogene ABL; Abelson strain of murine leukemia virus: ABL
ADA	12	102700	Adenosine deaminase	20q13.11	Adenosine deaminase; severe combined immunodeficiency due to adenosine deaminase deficiency; SCID due to ADA deficiency; ADA-SCID; ADA deficiency
APC	2, 8	175100	Adenomatous polyposis of the colon	5q21-q22	Familial polyposis of the colon: FPC; familial polyposis of the colon: FPC; familial adenomatous polyposis: FAP; Gardner syndrome: GS; adenomatous polyposis coli, attenuated: AAPC; 'deleted in polyposis' 2.5: DP2.5
APOE	9	107741	Apolipoprotein E	19q13.2	Apolipoprotein E, deficiency or defect of; hyperlipoproteinemia, type III; dysbetalipoproteinemia due to defect in apolipoprotein E-d; familial hyperbeta- and prebetalipoproteinemia; familial hypercholesterolemia with hyperlipemia; hyperlipemia with familial hypercholesterolemic xanthomatosis; broad-betalipoproteinemia; floating-betalipoproteinemia; coronary artery disease, severe, susceptibility to

GENE SYMBOL	CHAPTERS	OMIM[a] NUMBER	NAME	LOCATION	ALTERNATIVE TITLES AND SYMBOLS
APP	9	104760	Amyloid β-A4 precursor protein	21q21	Amyloid of aging and Alzheimer disease: AAA; cerebral vascular amyloid peptide: CVAP; protease nexin II: PN2; Alzheimer disease 1: AD1
AR	10	313700	Androgen receptor	Xq11-q12	Dihydrotestosterone receptor: DHTR
ATM	5	607585	Ataxia-telangiectasia mutated gene	11q22.3	
BCL2	11	151430	B-cell CLL, lymphoma 2	18q21.3	Oncogene B-cell leukemia 2; leukemia, chronic lymphatic, type 2; follicular lymphoma
BCL6	11	109565	B-cell lymphoma 6	3q27	Zinc finger protein 51: ZNF51; lymphoma-associated zinc finger gene on chromosome 3: LAZ3; BCL6/H4FM fusion gene; BCL6/Ikaros fusion gene; BCL6/LCP1 fusion gene; BCL6/IL21R fusion gene
BCR	8	151410	Breakpoint cluster region	22q11.21	BCR1; BCR/ABL fusion gene; BCR/FGFR1 fusion gene; BCR/PDGFRA fusion gene
BRCA1	5, 7, 8	113705	Breast cancer 1 gene	17q21	Breast cancer, type 1; breast cancer 1, early onset; breast-ovarian cancer
BRCA2	5, 7, 8	600185	Breast cancer 2 gene	13q12.3	Breast cancer, type 2; breast cancer 2, early-onset
CASP8	8	601763	Caspase 8, apoptosis-related cysteine protease	2q33-q34	MORT1-associated CED3 homolog: MACH; FADD-homologous ICE/CED3-like protease; FADD-like ICE: FLICE; MCH5
CCL3	11	182283	Chemokine, CC motif, ligand 3	17q11-q21	Small inducible cytokine A3, formerly: SCYA3; macrophage inflammatory protein 1-α: MIP1A; LD78-α
CCND2	11	123833	Cyclin D2	12p13	
CCR5	11	601373	Chemokine, CC motif, receptor 5	3p21	CC chemokine receptor 5: CCCKR5; CMKBR5; CKR5

GENE SYMBOL	CHAPTERS	OMIM[a] NUMBER	NAME	LOCATION	ALTERNATIVE TITLES AND SYMBOLS
CDKN2A	9	600160	Cyclin-dependent kinase inhibitor 2A	9p21	CDKN2; CDK4 inhibitor; multiple tumor suppressor 1: MTS1; TP16; p16(INK4); p16(INK4A); p19(ARF); p14(ARF)
CFTR	6, 9, 12	602421	Cystic fibrosis transmembrane conductance regulator	7q31.2	ATP-binding cassette, subfamily C, member 7: ABCC7
COL1A1	5 Web	120150	Collagen, type I, α-1	17q21.31-q22	Collagen of skin, tendon, and bone, α-1 chain; COL1A1/PDGFB fusion gene
COL1A2	5 Web	120160	Collagen, type I, α-2	7q22.1	Collagen of skin, tendon, and bone, α-2 chain
COL2A1	10	120140	Collagen, type II, α-1	12q13.11-q13.2	Collagen, type II; Collagen of cartilage; chondrocalcin; collagen, type XI, α-3, formerly: COL11A3; vitreoretinopathy with phalangeal epiphyseal dysplasia
CYP21A2	7	201910	Adrenal hyperplasia, congenital, due to 21-hydroxylase deficiency	6p21.3	Adrenal hyperplasia III; 21-hydroxylase deficiency; CYP21 deficiency; congenital adrenal hyperplasia 1: CAH1; cytochrome P450, subfamily XXIA, polypeptide 2: CYP21A2; cytochrome P450, subfamily XXI: CYP21; steroid cytochrome P450 21-hydroxylase: P450C21; 21-hydroxylase B: CYP21B; CA21H; cytochrome P450, subfamily XXIA, polypeptide 1 pseudogene: CYP21A1P; CYP21P; CYP21A; hyperandrogenism, non-classic type, due to 21-hydroxylase deficiency
CYP2C9	4, 11	601130	Cytochrome P450, subfamily IIC, polypeptide 9	10q24	
CYP2D	11	124030	Cytochrome P450, subfamily IID	22q13.1	P450DB1; debrisoquine 4-hydroxylase; debrisoquine hydroxylation; sparteine oxidation; nortriptyline oxidation; CYP2D6; CYP2D6L

GENE SYMBOL	CHAPTERS	OMIM[a] NUMBER	NAME	LOCATION	ALTERNATIVE TITLES AND SYMBOLS
CYP3A4	11	124010	Cytochrome P450, subfamily IIIA, polypeptide 4	7q22.1	CYP3; CYP3A; P450, family III; P450-III, steroid-inducible; glucocorticoid-inducible P450: P450C3; cytochrome P450PCN1; nifedipine oxidase
CYP3A5	11	605325	Cytochrome P450, subfamily IIIA, polypeptide 5	7q22.1	P450PCN3
DKK1	10	605189	Dickkopf, xenopus, homolog of, 1	10q11.2	
DM1	5	160900	Dystrophia myotonica 1	19q13.2–13.3	Dystrophia myotonica: DM; myotonic dystrophy 1; Steinert disease
DMPK	7	605377	Dystrophia myotonica protein kinase	19q13.2–13.3	DM kinase: DMK; DM protein kinase; myotonin–protein kinase
EDN3	9	131242	Endothelin 3	20q13.2–13.3	ET3
EDNRB	9	131244	Endothelin receptor, type B	13q22	Endothelin receptor, nonselective type: ETB; ETRB
ERBB2	8	164870	V-ERB-B2 avian erythroblastic leukemia viral oncogene homolog 2	17q21.1	Oncogene ERBB2; oncogene NGL, neuroblastoma- or glioblastoma-derived: NGL; NEU; tyrosine kinase-type cell surface receptor HER2: TKR1; herstatin
ERCC2	5	126340	Excision-repair, complementing defective, in Chinese hamster, 2	19q13.2–13.3	DNA repair defect EM9 of Chinese hamster ovary cells, complementation of: EM9
ERCC3	5	133510	Excision-repair, complementing defective, in Chinese hamster, 3	2q21	Xeroderma pigmentosum II: XP2; xeroderma pigmentosum, complementation group B: XPB; XP, group B; XPBC
ERCC4	5	133520	Excision-repair, complementing defective, in Chinese hamster, 4	16p13.3-p13.13	
ERCC5	5	133530	Excision-repair, complementing defective, in Chinese hamster, 5	13q33	ERCM2; UV damage, excision repair of, UV-135: UVDR; ultraviolet sensitivity, mouse, complementation of; RAD2, yeast, homolog of; xeroderma pigmentosum, group G correcting protein: XPGC; XPG; xeroderma pigmentosum/Cockayne syndrome complex: XPG/CS

GENE SYMBOL	CHAPTERS	OMIM[a] NUMBER	NAME	LOCATION	ALTERNATIVE TITLES AND SYMBOLS
FANCD1	5	605724	Fanconi anemia, complementation group D1	13q12.3	FAD1
FGF1	12	131220	Fibroblast growth factor 1	5q31	Endothelial cell growth factor: ECGF; heparin-binding growth factor 1: HBGF1; fibroblast growth factor, acidic: FGFA; endothelial cell growth factor, α: ECGFA; endothelial cell growth factor, β: ECGFB
FGF4	12	164980	Fibroblast growth factor 4	11q13	Heparin secretory transforming protein 1: HSTF1; oncogene HST; human stomach cancer, transforming factor from; FGF-related oncogene; Kaposi sarcoma oncogene: KFGF
FGFR3	7	134934	Fibroblast growth factor receptor 3	4p16.3	
FMR1	5	309550	Fragile site mental retardation 1 gene	Xq27.3	Fragile X mental retardation protein: FMRP; fragile X syndrome; fragile X mental retardation syndrome; mental retardation, X-linked, associated with marXq28; X-linked mental retardation and macro-orchidism; marker X syndrome; Martin-Bell syndrome; fragile site, folic acid type, rare, FRA(X)(q27.3): FRAXA; fragile X tremor/ataxia syndrome: FXTAS
FN1	11	135600	Fibronectin 1	2q34	FN; large, external, transformation-sensitive protein: LETS; FNZ
G6PD	7	305900	Glucose-6-phosphate dehydrogenase	Xq28	Anemia, nonspherocytic hemolytic, due to G6PD deficiency
GATA1	10	305371	GATA-binding protein 1	Xp11.23	Erythroid transcription factor 1: ERYF1; globin transcription factor 1: GF1; transcription factor GATA1; leukemia, megakaryoblastic, of Down syndrome
GATA2	10	137295	GATA-binding protein 2	3	
GATA3	10	131320	GATA-binding protein 3	10p15	Enhancer-binding protein GATA3
GATA4	10	600576	GATA-binding protein 4	8p23.1-p22	

GENE SYMBOL	CHAPTERS	OMIM[a] NUMBER	NAME	LOCATION	ALTERNATIVE TITLES AND SYMBOLS
GCK	9	138079	Glucokinase	7p15-p13	GK; GLK; hexokinase 4: HK4
GDNF	9	600837	Glial cell line–derived neurotrophic factor	5p13.1-p12	
GNAS1	5	139320	GNAS complex locus	20q13.2	Guanine nucleotide-binding protein, α-stimulating activity polypeptide 1: GNAS1; Gs, α-subunit; stimulatory G protein; adenylate cyclase stimulatory protein, α-subunit; secretogranin VI; neuroendocrine secretory protein 55: NESP55; XL-α-S: XLAS
H19	4	103280	H19 gene	11p15.5	Adult skeletal muscle gene: ASM; ASM1; D11S813E
HFE	7 web	235200	Hemochromatosis	6p21.3	HLAH; hemochromatosis, hereditary: HH; hemochromatosis gene: HFE
HNF4A	9	600281	Hepatocyte nuclear factor 4-α	20q12-q13.1	HNF4-α; hepatocyte nuclear factor 4: HNF4; transcription factor 14, hepatic nuclear factor: TCF14
HOXA13	10	142959	Homeobox A13	7p15-p14.2	Homeobox 1J: HOX1J
HOXD13	10	142989	Homeobox D13	2q31-q32	Homeobox 4I: HOX4I
IKBKG	7	300248	Inhibitor of κ-light polypeptide gene enhancer in B cells, kinase of, γ	Xq28	IKK-γ; NF-κ-B essential modulator: NEMO; FIP3
IL2RG	12	308380	Interleukin 2 receptor, γ	Xq13	CD132 antigen: CD132
JAG1	5	601920	Jagged 1	20p12	JAGL1; deafness, congenital heart defects, and posterior embryotoxon
KCNQ1	5	607542	Potassium channel, voltage-gated, KQT-like subfamily, member 1	11p15.5	KVLQT1; potassium channel, voltage-gated, Shaker-related subfamily, member 9: KCNA9; KCNA8
KCNQ1OT1	4	604115	KCNQ1-overlapping transcript 1	11p15.5	Long QT intronic transcript 1: LIT1

GENE SYMBOL	CHAPTERS	OMIM[a] NUMBER	NAME	LOCATION	ALTERNATIVE TITLES AND SYMBOLS
LHCGR	10	152790	Luteinizing hormone, choriogonadotropin receptor	2p21	Lutropin-choriogonadotropin receptor: LCGR; gonadotropin receptor; gonadotropin unresponsiveness; Leydig cell hypoplasia; Leydig cell agenesis; Leydig cell adenoma
LMO2	11,12	180385	LIM domain only 2	11p13	Rhombotin 2: RBTN2; rhombotin-like 1: RBTNL1, RHOM2; T-cell translocation gene 2: TTG2
MADH4	8	600993	Mothers against decapentaplegic, Drosophila, homolog of, 4	18q21.1	SMA- AND MAD-related protein 4: SMAD4; deleted in pancreatic carcinoma 4: DPC4
MC1R	9	155555	Melanocortin 1 receptor	16q24.3	Melanocyte-stimulating hormone receptor: MSHR; melanotropin receptor
MECP2	4	300005	Methyl-CpG-binding protein 2	Xq28	Encephalopathy, nonprogressive, neonatal onset
MEF2A	9	600660	MADS box transcription enhancer factor 2, polypeptide A	15q26	
MET	8	164860	MET proto-oncogene	7q31	Oncogene MET; hepatocyte growth factor receptor: HGFR; renal cell carcinoma, papillary, 2 gene: RCCP2
MITF	9 web	156845	Microphthalmia-associated transcription factor	3p14.1–12.3	Microphthalmia, mouse, homolog of; MITF-A; MITF-C; MITF-H; MITF-M
MLH1	5,8	120436	Colon cancer, familial nonpolyposis, type 2	3p21.3	FCC2; COCA2; colorectal cancer, hereditary nonpolyposis, type 2: HNPCC2; MutL, *E. coli*, homolog of, 1: MLH1
MSH2	5,8	120435	Colon cancer, familial nonpolyposis, type 1	2p22-p21	FCC1; COCA1; colorectal cancer, hereditary nonpolyposis, type 1: HNPCC1; HNPCC; MutS, *E. coli*, homolog of, 2: MSH2
MSH6	5,8	600678	MutS, *E. coli*, homolog of, 6	2p16	G/T mismatch-binding protein: GTBP; colorectal cancer, hereditary nonpolyposis, type 5: HNPCC5

GENE SYMBOL	CHAPTERS	OMIM[a] NUMBER	NAME	LOCATION	ALTERNATIVE TITLES AND SYMBOLS
MTHFD1	9	172460	Methylenetetrahydrofolate dehydrogenase 1	14q24	Methylenetetrahydrofolate dehydrogenase, methenyltetrahydrofolate cyclohydrolase, formyltetrahydrofolate synthetase, NADP(+) dependent; methyltetrahydrofolate cyclohydrolase deficiency
MTHFR	9	607093	5,10-Methylenetetrahydrofolate reductase	1p36.3	
MYCN	8	164840	V-MYC avian myelocytomatosis viral-related oncogene, neuroblastoma-derived	2p24.1	Oncogene NMYC; NMYC oncogene; avian myelocytomatosis viral-related oncogene, neuroblastoma-derived; neuroblastoma MYC oncogene
NF1	7	162200	Neurofibromatosis, type I	17q11.2	Neurofibromatosis; Von Recklinghausen disease; neurofibromin; neurofibromatosis, type, with leukemia; neurofibromatosis, type 1, with glioma
NKX2.5	10	600584	NK2, Drosophila, homolog of, E	5q34	Cardiac-specific homeobox: CSX; NKX2.5, mouse, homolog of
NR0B1	10	300473	Nuclear receptor subfamily 0, group B, member 1	Xp21.3-p21.2	DSS-AHC critical region on the X chromosome 1, gene 1: DAX1
NRTN	9	602018	Neurturin	19p13.3	NTN
OTC	12	300461	Ornithine carbamoyltransferase	Xp21.1	Ornithine transcarbamylase
PAX3	9 web	606597	Paired box gene 3	2q35	Paired domain gene HuP2: HUP2; PAX3/FKHR fusion gene
PMS1	5,8	600258	Postmeiotic segregation increased, S. cerevisiae, 1	2q31-q33	Mismatch repair gene PMSL1: PMSL1; colorectal cancer, hereditary nonpolyposis, type 3: HNPCC3
PMS2	5,8	600259	Postmeiotic segregation increased, S. cerevisiae, 2	7p22	Mismatch repair gene PMSL2: colorectal cancer, hereditary nonpolyposis, type: HNPCC4

GENE SYMBOL	CHAPTERS	OMIM[a] NUMBER	NAME	LOCATION	ALTERNATIVE TITLES AND SYMBOLS
PPARG	9	601487	Peroxisome proliferator-activated receptor-γ	3p25	PPARG1; PPARG2; PPARG3; PAX8/PPARG fusion gene
PSEN1	9	104311	Presenilin 1	14q24.3	PS1; S182
PSEN2	9	600759	Presenilin 2	1q31-q42	PS2; STM2
PTCH	10	601309	Patched, Drosophila, homolog of	9q22.3	PTC; holoprosencephaly 7: HPE7
PTEN	8	601728	Phosphatase and tensin homolog	10q23.31	PTEN1; mutated in multiple advanced cancers 1: MMAC1; phosphatase and tensin homolog deleted on chromosome 10
RB1	8	180200	Retinoblastoma	13q14.1-q14.2	RB; osteosarcoma, retinoblastoma-related; p105-Rb
RECQL3	2,5	604610	RECQ protein-like 3	15q26.1	DNA helicase, RECQ-like, type 2: RECQ2; Bloom syndrome gene: BLM
RET	5,7,8,9	164761	Rearranged during transfection proto-oncogene	10q11.2	RET proto-oncogene; RET/ELKS fusion gene
SHH	10	600725	Sonic hedgehog	7q36	
SIX3	10	603714	Sine oculis homeobox, Drosophila, homolog of, 3	2p21	
SOX10	9	602229	SRY-BOX 10	22q13	SRY-related HMG-BOX gene 10; dominant megacolon, mouse, homolog of: DOM
SOX9	10	608160	SRY-BOX 9	17q24.3-q25.1	SRY-related HMG-BOX gene 9; sex reversal, autosomal, 1: SRA1
SPINK1	9	167790	Serine protease inhibitor, KAZAL-type, 1	5q32	Pancreatic secretory trypsin inhibitor: PSTI; tumor-associated trypsin inhibitor: TATI
SRY	10	480000	Sex-determining region Y	Yp11.3	Testis-determining factor: TDF; testis-determining factor on Y: TDY
TAL1	12	187040	T-cell acute lymphocytic leukemia 1	1p32	Stem cell leukemia hematopoietic transcription factor: SCL; T-cell leukemia/lymphoma 5: TCL5

GENE SYMBOL	CHAPTERS	OMIM[a] NUMBER	NAME	LOCATION	ALTERNATIVE TITLES AND SYMBOLS
TBX1	10	602054	T-BOX 1	22q11.2	
TBX5	10	601620	T-BOX 5	12q24.1	
TGIF	10	602630	Transforming growth factor-β-induced factor	18p11.3	TGFB-induced factor; TG-interacting factor
TP53	5,8	191170	Tumor protein p53	17p13.1	P53; transformation-related protein 53: TRP53; colon tumors, concurrent multiple primary
UBE3A	4	601623	Ubiquitin-protein ligase E3A	15q11-q13	Human papillomavirus E6-associated protein: E6AP
UGT1A1	7	191740	UDP-glycosyltransferase 1 family, polypeptide A1	2q37	Uridine diphosphate glycosyltransferase 1 family, polypeptide A1; uridine diphosphate glycosyl transferase 1: UGT1; UDP-glycosyl transferase 1; uridine diphosphate glucurono syltransferase, bilirubin/phenol; phenol/biliru bin UDP-glucuronosyltransferase; GNT1
VEGF	12	192240	Vascular endothelial growth factor	6p12	VEGFA
WT1	10	607102	Wilms tumor 1 gene	11p13	
XIST	4	314670	X inactivation-specific transcript	Xq13.2	X inactivation center, included: XIC
XPA	5	278700	Xeroderma pigmentosum, complementation group A	9q22.3	XP, group A; xeroderma pigmentosum I: XP1; XPA correcting; XPA complementing: XPAC; XPA gene
XPC	5	278720	Xeroderma pigmentosum, complementation group C	3p25	XPCC; XP, group C; xeroderma pigmentosum III: XP3; XPC gene
ZIC2	10	603073	Zinc finger protein of cerebellum, 2	13q32	ZIC family member 2; holoprosencephaly 5: HPE5
ZNF9	7	116955	Zinc finger protein 9	3q13.3-q24	Cellular retroviral nucleic acid-binding protein 1: CNBP1

[a]OMIM = Online Mendelian Inheritance in Man. www.ncbi.nlm.nih.gov/omim

Index

Page numbers in *italic* denote figures; page numbers followed by "t" denote tables; page numbers followed by "b" denote boxes.